CONNECTING

Raising Kids in the Digital World

Megan Moreno, MD, MSEd, MPH, FAAP
Jenny Radesky, MD, FAAP

American Academy of Pediatrics
DEDICATED TO THE HEALTH OF ALL CHILDREN®

American Academy of Pediatrics Publishing Staff
Jeff Mahony, *Senior Director, Professional and Consumer Publishing*
Kathryn Sparks, *Senior Editor, Consumer Publishing*
Annika Hawkinson, *Editorial Assistant*
Shannan Martin, *Production Manager, Consumer Publications*
Amanda Helmholz, *Medical Copy Editor*
Soraya Alem, *Manager, Digital Publishing*
Sara Hoerdeman, *Marketing and Acquisitions Manager, Consumer Products*

Published by the American Academy of Pediatrics
345 Park Blvd
Itasca, IL 60143
630/626-6000
www.aap.org

The American Academy of Pediatrics is an organization of 67,000 primary care pediatricians, pediatric medical subspecialists, and pediatric surgical specialists dedicated to the health, safety, and well-being of all infants, children, adolescents, and young adults.

Printed in the United States of America

9-537 1 2 3 4 5 6 7 8 9 10
CB0146
ISBN: 978-1-61002-889-9
eBook: 978-1-61002-891-2
EPUB: 978-1-61002-890-5

Cover and publication design by R. Scott Rattray
Jenny Radesky photograph © Nell Boss Photography.

Library of Congress Control Number: 2025948848

What People Are Saying About *Connecting*

Connecting: Raising Kids in the Digital World is the book that should be in the hands of every parent doing that interesting challenging job in this rapidly changing environment. Drs Moreno and Radesky will be the lucid explainers, and the sympathetic guides and companions that parents need at their sides—as do their kids.

Perri Klass, MD, FAAP, national medical director, Reach Out and Read

Most parents feel like we're doing it wrong when it comes to kids and technology. In *Connecting,* pediatricians and leading researchers Drs Megan Moreno and Jenny Radesky reveal that "there is more than one right way to parent around technology." Even better, their book is designed to help you find *your* version of "right"—one that, it turns out, will bring you closer to the kids you love. *Connecting* is an invitation for the generation of parents who are ready to trade anxiety and guilt for intentional strategies that are grounded in deep research and backed by decades of real-world clinical experience.

Emily Weinstein, EdD, coauthor of *Behind Their Screens: What Teens Are Facing (and Adults Are Missing),* principal investigator and codirector of the Center for Digital Thriving at Harvard Graduate School of Education

Connecting is the timely new book every parent needs. Drawing on the latest science, 2 of the leading researchers on children and screen time cut through the noise with practical wisdom on how to ensure kids have healthy development in all areas of their lives while becoming critical thinkers about what they encounter online. I wholeheartedly recommend this book!

Delaney Ruston, MD, filmmaker of the Screenagers series, author of *Parenting in the Screen Age: A Guide for Calm Conversations*

Since I'm a pediatrician and supposed expert in kids and media, you might think I had all the answers when raising my own 5 kids. What I had instead was even more questions. And the people I went to for answers were my friends and colleagues, Dr Megan Moreno and Dr Jenny Radesky. Now you, too, can access their wisdom just by opening a book! "Connect" with this resource, and keep your kids connected to the world.

David L. Hill, MD, FAAP, author of *Dad to Dad: Parenting Like a Pro;* clinical professor of pediatrics, Seattle Children's Hospital

Every week, I talk with storytellers, researchers, and families about helping kids thrive in today's media world. *Connecting* is one of the most balanced and practical guides I've read, translating excellent science into advice parents can actually use.

Yalda T. Uhls, MBA, PhD, founder of the Center for Scholars & Storytellers at UCLA, developmental psychologist and former media executive, parent

Dedication

This book is for our families.

CONTENTS

PART 4: Risky Behaviors

ACKNOWLEDGMENTS

We are grateful to have the opportunity to share what we know and have learned about healthy media use and families through this book. First and foremost, we are appreciative of the input and expertise of our American Academy of Pediatrics (AAP) editor, Kathryn Sparks. We are also thankful to Sara Hoerdeman for providing the opportunity and inspiration for this work. We want to express our utmost appreciation for the insights and knowledge of our colleagues at the AAP Center of Excellence on Social Media and Youth Mental Health, including its leaders Nicole Owings-Fonner, Ashley Horne, and Julie Gorzkowski, as well as input from the Youth Advisory Panel led by Marija Hegel and Molly Moynihan. We have both benefited and learned from the expertise of our colleagues in 2 AAP committees, the Council on Communications and Media and the Council on Adolescents and Young Adults, and are thankful for these pediatrician colleagues and their expertise.

We sought input from a variety of parents and topic experts during the writing of this book to ensure that the content represented parents' lived experiences and met with recommendations from experts. To recognize the individual contributions of these incredible reviewers, we would like to list them by name, including the following: Erin Ryan, Sushant Srinivasan, Ryan McAdams, Chelsea Olson, Christine Richards, Reva Finkelman, Abbey Granger, Holly Gerla, Michelle Kelly, Faith Portier, Leigh Fredericks, Jess Babal, Jeff Yaeger, Kerry Gannon-Loew, Hannah Wakefield, Kerri LeBlanc, Sophie Brickman, and, last but never least, Ande Jones.

We wouldn't be the researchers and doctors we are without the love and patience of our families. We are grateful for our own children and partners who have taught us the importance of connecting both with and without technology.

Finally, we would like to thank our patients and their families whom we have seen in clinic over many years, as well as youth and families who have shared their experiences and expertise with us through our research. This book is in honor of you.

INTRODUCTION

If parenting around technology feels challenging to you—congratulations, join the club of millions of other parents! Parents say that raising children today feels more challenging than at any time in recent history and that technology is a big contributor to that stress.

As pediatricians and medical directors of a national center that focuses on media and youth, we have talked to thousands of families about the challenges of tech-life balance in today's world. As parents, we have felt these challenges too. Compared with the childhoods that we might have had or that our parents had, childhood now involves literally being in contact with computers, the internet, or digital technology through most of our waking hours. Our job as parents now includes helping kids navigate an increasingly complex—and rapidly changing—digital world.

When we use the word *parents* in this book, we mean the main caregiver for a child—this could be the child's biological parents, adopted parents, grandparents, or other legal guardian. If you love and care for a kid, this book is for you.

However, *screen time doesn't occur in a vacuum*. There are multiple factors, such as our stress levels, the availability of child care or after-school programs, or a family's communication patterns that influence how technology is used and what effect it has on us. This book will help you navigate devices, social media, video gaming, and AI with your kids while acknowledging these other factors and offering skills for how to feel more connected in your family relationships. Because secure relationships are the bedrock of child and adult mental health, the guidance in this book will always come back to how to support relationships; avoid power struggles; and carve out time for family, peers, and offline experiences and how to choose technology that supports real connection and mental well-being.

There are a few reasons why parenting around technology feels hard. Understanding these foundational concepts can normalize the way you are feeling and help you work around these barriers (which are not your fault). It is common for us as parents to immediately blame ourselves, but this is a complex issue with a lot of layers. Parents, we are simply the layer closest to our kids.

The Polarization Problem

The public conversation about kids and technology is *way* too intense and often judgmental. This is because people are anxious when new technologies disrupt our usual ways of living, and the current disruption is faster than prior ones have been. However, it may be helpful to know that there were similar panics in the past about TV in the 1950s and the telephone in the 1920s. New technologies often spark these feelings of excitement, fear, panic, and outrage across our society.

Over the past few years, headlines have been full of claims that smartphones and social media are the cause of all youth mental health problems, as well as claims that it's all an overblown moral panic. The truth is somewhere in the middle: Modern technologies have been rapidly introduced without designing them in ways that support child or teen well-being, and this has caused harm in many kids. It's also true that many kids and parents derive social support and joy from technologies, thus finding it difficult to completely avoid a digital world that is so enmeshed with our livelihoods and culture. Effects of media vary by children's strengths and challenges, developmental stage, and how much social support they have from parents and schools offline. These types of explanations that involve complexity—rather than all-or-nothing choices—often don't trend in sound bites on social media, so you might not see them as much.

> Our goal is to take the temperature down on this conversation, talk in a way that centers youth development and family relationships, and be as pragmatic as possible. We want you to feel less anxious—not more—when you finish this book.

When Parenting Feels Like a Competitive Sport

The other reason for judgment in public conversations about children and technology is that our society, built on ideals of individualism and pull-yourself-up-by-your-bootstraps self-reliance, often expects *individuals* to manage problems that the *larger society created.* Unfortunately, when something does go wrong, at home, at school, or with an individual child, the parents always are the ones who get blamed. In a society where competition starts prenatally—from a child care spot all the way to a college admission—we may not question our culture's preoccupation with cultivating and optimizing children. And if you are trying to live up to that perfect ideal, you may feel anxious and not good enough. It will constantly make you feel the need to judge yourself against some external standard. The reasons for this competitive culture are deep-seated and include

1. Living in a society that doesn't provide as many parenting supports as other industrialized nations, like parental leave or child care, so we feel like we are competing for scarce resources
2. Being subject to marketing in the United States that has long tried to convince parents (mothers especially) that their child is "at risk" without whatever product or service is for sale
3. Being bombarded by messages in the news that often tap into this idea of risk because it evokes emotion in us, such as fears of loss or shame, which encourage us to click or watch longer and which can shape the norms of how we think about parenting

But parenting is not a competition to be won. It's a process. In this book, we come from the standpoint that parents are trying their best and that there are many ways to parent around technology in a healthy way. This is important enough that we'll say it twice: *There is more than one right way to parent around technology.* We show examples of these different approaches in each chapter, highlighting what you can try anywhere from a screen-free to a tech-embracing strategy.

As parents, you have navigated this "more than one right way" before. As parents of infants, you discovered there is more than one right way to get your baby to sleep through the night (although Megan would offer that there was a period in which it felt like her son wouldn't sleep no matter what she tried). As parents of toddlers, you discovered there is more than one way to potty train. You have been here before. In fact, a 20th-century British pediatrician and psychoanalyst, Donald Winnicott, coined a term we love, the "good enough" parent, observing that parents don't need to meet some impossible "perfect" standard to raise a healthy child—there is a lot of room for variation and learning from failure. In fact, parents *shouldn't* strive for perfection because they'll wind up overdoing it and not leaving enough room for the child to figure out who they are and what they can do on their own. Accepting the idea of being good enough also removes the pressure to be "right" all the time—it leaves space for you to learn as a parent and grow as a person.

Instead of trying to perform against some cultural brand of perfect parenting, parents tell us it's helpful to *re-center their goals around who their child is*—not who our society sees as "perfect" or "optimal"—and to start trusting themselves. In fact, we work with many families raising neurodivergent children who have found grace and relief in the process of stepping out of the competitive-parent, child-optimizing rat race and learning to focus on their unique child and their family relationships instead.

Perfect parent versus good enough parent

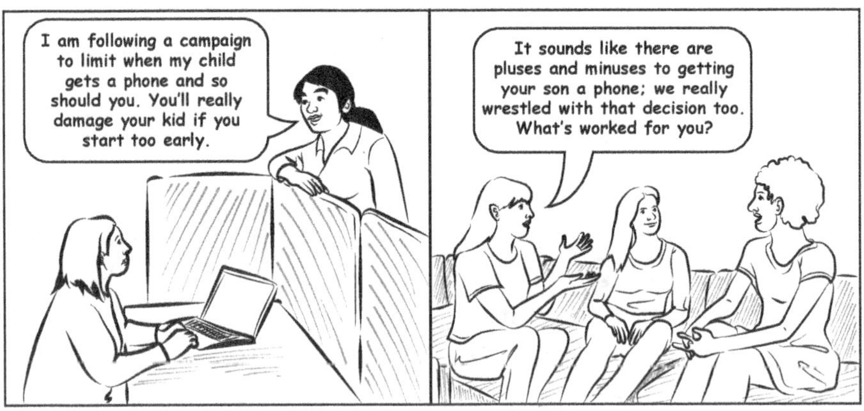
I am following a campaign to limit when my child gets a phone and so should you. You'll really damage your kid if you start too early.
It sounds like there are pluses and minuses to getting your son a phone; we really wrestled with that decision too. What's worked for you?

The Engagement-Optimized Internet

The last reason it is hard to parent around technology is that modern technology has exploded around us at a pace that society hasn't experienced before. Older technologies such as the TV or telephone took decades to fully saturate US households. In contrast, the iPad took only 80 days, and *Pokémon Go* took 19 days to reach 50 million global users. This means that, from generation to generation, we don't have as much shared understanding of how to live around these technologies and use them in ways that augment our lives. We don't have an intuitive understanding of how to teach our children about technology in the way we know how to teach them to scramble an egg or ride a bike.

But many tech investors want superfast growth—they make more rapid returns on their investments when technology "grows fast and breaks things"—usually without thinking about how kids will use these products. As the 2026 American Academy of Pediatrics media guidelines discussed, technology designs that meet the goals of quarterly earnings calls—such as features that keep users scrolling longer so that they watch more ads—can often work against our goals as parents, like helping our anxious child get a good night's sleep. We describe these designs and their underlying moneymaking purpose throughout this book in a section called the "Tech Corner." Here we will suggest different ways the tech world could be designed better. The goal is to build your digital literacy so that you can recognize these designs, discuss them with your kids, avoid products that contain them, and turn off certain functions linked to these designs.

The digital world is a *lot* right now. Does that mean you and your family should avoid it altogether? The truth is even if you prefer to keep your household relatively low-tech, you'll probably need to use computers and devices in some way for managing your job and life, and your kids may be provided devices to use in school. And there's a lot of joy, laughs, and inspiration to find online, so no matter what your style is when it comes to tech in your household, this book aims to share the basics of how to guide your family in healthy balance. We try to role model a mindset of healthy skepticism or experimentation about trying out new devices, games, or apps. With shame and judgment removed from the conversation, this book will help you have regular conversations with your children to coach them in things such as finding good online content, understanding online privacy, building self-control, and recognizing nonsense when they see it.

In fact, that's why we titled this book *Connecting*—to show that parenting around technology is an ongoing, imperfect, and skill-building process that actually can help you understand your child better. We thought about naming it *Connected*, but that would imply that there's an end point, something to check off your list...but sorry, parenting just isn't like that.

How to Use This Book

In this book, we use our experience as pediatricians, parents, and researchers to share the best tips we have as if we were talking to a family or patient in our clinic. Each chapter is centered on a health topic or a developmental process. We mention specific technologies at times, but we focus more on design features of technologies (eg, Does it have a feed? Does it allow chatting with others? Does it have an AI component?) in the hope that despite inevitable technological advances, this book will still be relevant in 10 years. This topic is complicated, so to help make that complexity more digestible, we include graphics in each chapter.

Definition: This icon indicates a definition of a major or complex concept.

Key Point: This icon indicates a key concept that you can keep in mind when making decisions about technology use.

Tech Corner: These sections describe how technology design or the culture of digital spaces affects a particular issue.

Research Corner: If you like digging more into the research, these sections include a description of a relevant research study, including Megan's or Jenny's previous studies.

Practical Takeaway: This icon indicates a practical strategy to try that is based on the research and ideas that the chapter offered.

Conversation Tips: These tips provide concrete ideas for how to talk about the topic with your children or teens.

We also focus on how to listen to our children and understand what they need at different developmental stages. Unlike public messaging that often positions kids as victims, our focus is to see them as incredible sources of ideas and passion. To truly help kids when they struggle, we need to meet them in a space of understanding, see things from their perspective, and offer support with healthy limits that help them solve problems and learn from the experience. When we micromanage or throw our hands up when they struggle, this developmental progress is less likely to happen, and it will be more difficult to launch kids into independence when they turn 18.

At the end of each chapter, we summarize the main points in a section called "Connecting the Dots," which suggests a few ideas about how to apply the main points of the chapter to your everyday life. We know that just reading a book isn't going to help as much as living it. Therefore, we suggest ideas for how to try 1 or 2 of the following:

- An experiment you can try in order to shift your family's habits. Being a good enough parent means learning as you go. We recommend a few simple ideas for trying to change your family's tech habits for a few weeks.
- How to talk to your child or teen about the topic. Technology can be a cringe-inducing topic. We suggest a few conversation starters or ideas to bounce off your older children and teens.
- How to talk to your friends or neighbors about the topic. Parents often feel isolated and judged about technology and screen use, yet so many of us are going through similar things. We suggest a

few topics to discuss with friends the next time you grab coffee together, host a playdate, or see each other at school pickup.

We recognize that books have limitations. You live a busy life, so we wrote this book to be read in bite-size amounts that you can try to apply to everyday life. Also, we have never met you. When we give guidance in our clinics, we base it on the relationship and trust we build with our patient and their family. Our discussions are never one-size-fits-all. There is nuance. It depends on the child and parents who are sitting in front of us and their unique strengths and challenges. To make this a book that feels like it speaks to everyone, we include a few vignettes, as well as comic strip–like examples of the dos and don'ts of talking to family members about tech, and highlight the ways children and teens with different levels of anxiety, attention problems, social skills struggles, or other neurodivergent differences can have particular relationships with media.

We recommend that you start with Part 1, Relationships. Family and peer relationships are the bedrock of how children build resilience and healthy emotional development and how you can understand what they are going through. Then you can either read through the rest of the book or select chapters according to your current interests or concerns. Part 2 focuses on healthy behaviors such as sleep, physical activity, nutrition, and learning; Part 3 focuses on mental and emotional well-being and the different ways technology can affect it; and Part 4 dives into risky behaviors. We want this to be a book that you can refer back to as your child grows older or struggles with new things. Our goal is to help you learn from that friction, not avoid it or blame yourself. Key topics and principles are bolded throughout the book, so if you want some advice on a particular technological issue such as influencers, parental controls, or misinformation, you can find the definitions easily.

Thanks for joining us on this journey of connecting.

Part 1 | **Relationships**

Chapter 1

FAMILY RELATIONSHIPS

What we will cover

- Important parenting concepts relevant to technology, including "looking under the hood" of your child's behavior (see Parenting Like a Good Enough Parent section later in this chapter), how to find the sweet spot of autonomy support, and how to treat struggles as learning experiences
- How technology can be a disconnector in family relationships and how to prevent this
- How tech designs keep us on devices longer than we planned
- How technology can be a connector in family relationships and how to support this
- What to do if you are struggling to connect with your child

Parent-child relationships are the most important thing in a child's life. (As a reminder, when we use the word *parents* in this book, we mean the main caregiver(s) for a child—this could be the child's biological parents, adopted parents, grandparents, or other legal guardian.) What's frustrating about modern parenting culture is that we are often taught to worry about all the ways we might mess up rather than seeing and embracing the enormous opportunity that comes with being such a strong force of love and support in our child's life.

Parents tell us that they struggle with *how* to be this powerful source of love and support. Children don't come with an owner's manual on how to keep them mentally healthy, how to respond to their emotions, or how to be a good enough parent—a lot is intuition. Some of this intuition is based on what we were given during our own childhoods—how our own parents parented. Many parents of our patients tell us that they want to avoid re-creating parenting behaviors they experienced as a child such as lay-it-on-thick guilt trips, yelling and overreacting to small problems, excessive alcohol use, or swallowing of emotions. The more we understand these types of upstream drivers of our parenting behaviors, the more we can act with intention rather than with automatic emotional reactions. In this chapter, we unpack important parent-child relationship concepts related to technology and how to use them.

Parenting Like a Good Enough Parent

Being good enough means being there for kids and showing them that we can handle tough moments together. These distressful moments may start with an infant crying and knowing they have a parent who will pick them up, a kindergartner trusting that their caregiver will be there to pick them up after school and ask about their day, or a teenager knowing that their caregiver will listen to them and not overreact (or at least try not to) when they mess up at school and need advice. These types of daily interactions help kids build an understanding of themselves and feel OK being vulnerable with other people (which helps them be better parents and partners when they get older).

You might think these examples all set a low bar for parenting, but maybe that is because we are constantly told by our culture that the following make a good parent:

- Your child is always happy (not possible).
- You are immediately responsive to every child's need (not necessary or possible).
- You buy your child whatever they want (not actually good for kids).
- You prevent your child from experiencing any type of risk or disappointment (also not good for kids).
- Your child never experiences pain or hurt feelings (not realistic).

Instead, the most important parts of a healthy parent-child relationship that you'll hear us talk about in this chapter and the rest of book include the following:

- **Trying to understand your child.** In developmental psychology, this is called *mind-mindedness*—but we also call it "looking under the hood." It means that caregivers wonder about what's going on in that little brain: Why did they do that? What are they struggling with? This isn't always easy—kids throw a lot of bizarre behavior at their parents. But it's a lot easier to help a child through a problem when you wonder about the *struggle behind the behavior* and not simply react to the behavior. This often requires the parent to be calm and have enough mental bandwidth to wonder what their child is feeling. In other words, when you have 5 million things on your mind, or are dealing with your own stress, it's harder to pause, open your mind, and try to take in your child's perspective. However, it really pays off. Again and again, we find that when our patients feel understood, they in turn are calmer and can learn to identify and manage their emotions better.
- **Finding the sweet spot of *autonomy support*.** This means helping your child do things with hints and light help, where you scaffold them—not micromanage or spoon-feed them—and not being hands-off and saying, "Build it yourself; I'm busy!" Allow kids to try things with a little of your support—they learn best from planning it themselves and recalibrating when they experience failure. Research from the Early Head Start Research and Evaluation Project published in 2023 showed that autonomy-supportive parenting helps younger kids be ready to handle the new cognitive challenges of kindergarten, mostly through building self-regulation skills. Similarly, teens whose parents support their emotional development with autonomy support (understanding, warmth, and limits) have lower rates of anxiety and depression. Autonomy support helps kids become independent problem-solvers and copers. Table 1.1 provides examples of what scaffolding looks like in everyday experiences.

- **Embracing the concept of *repair*.** This means accepting that as a parent you will mess up. But you'll learn from it. Repair acknowledges that parents are going to misunderstand and mess up with their kids much of the time, but if you can come back together when things calm down, connect emotionally, and talk through the problem, your bond will be even stronger. And you will be teaching your child as you go.

Table 1.1 | **Scaffolding at Different Ages**

Child's Age and Activity Example	*Micromanaging/ Control*	*Scaffolding*	*Hands-Off/Providing No Help*
Early childhood: Trying to figure out a new puzzle	Putting the puzzle pieces together yourself instead of the child doing it	Showing how to put a couple puzzle pieces together, then giving hints like showing the child how to turn pieces around	Telling a child to do the puzzle on their own
School years: Asking for help with math homework	Giving them the homework answers	Asking, "How did your teacher show you to solve those problems?"	Saying, "I don't remember any math; I can't help."
Adolescence: Worrying about a negative peer interaction at school	Emailing the teacher or calling the peer's parent to fix the situation, or telling the child exactly what to do	Asking, "Why do you think they did that? How did you handle it? How would you handle it next time?"	Dismissing the teen's concerns, for example, saying, "Bullies will always be like that."

Technology Can Be a Disconnector or a Connector

Now that we've covered the general components of a healthy parent-child relationship, let's think about how technology interacts with these relationships. One way to think about this is whether technology acts as a disconnector or a connector within the family.

Tech as a Disconnector: Technoference

Before the introduction of BlackBerry phones and smartphones in the 2000s, TVs pretty much stayed where they were set up, and computers needed time to boot up and connect to the internet. But once smartphones and then tablets burst onto the scene, there was an array of different ways parents or children could use media in any room of the house or car at any time. In my (Jenny) interviews with parents in the 2010s through 2020, parents found this time both exciting and completely exhausting. Email and news of the world could reach them instantaneously. People could find them through text or social media whenever they wanted, and privacy felt like a concept of the past. This introduced a new kind of challenge for parents—toggling between the emotional work of parenting and all of the stimuli on their phones. Parents even disclosed that it was a relief when they had a power outage and they couldn't access the internet—and they could instead "single-task" on family.

Definitions

The use of phones to escape from social interactions is called **phubbing** (phone + snubbing) or **technoference** (technology + interference). In research conducted all over the globe, researchers have found that when parents pay attention to technology, they interact less with their children and are less responsive; therefore, they are less mind-minded about their children and have a harder time managing child behavior.

Parents' own use of technology has been an area I (Jenny) have studied extensively. In a 2018 study, my collaborator Brandon McDaniel followed 183 couples raising young children for 6 months. Every few months, he asked the parents to complete surveys about technoference (the frequency of tech device use during parent-child time), their parenting stress, and their child's behavior. We found that more technoference predicts worse child behavior over time, suggesting that when parent-child activities are disrupted by technology, crucial social-emotional learning moments are being displaced, and when parents are looking at their phones, their kids may act out to get more attention. Yet the interesting finding in this study was that difficult child behavior *also predicted* technoference over time. We interpreted this—as backed up by parent interviews—as evidence that parents often escape from cranky kids by using their phones. Parents may want to "check one thing" or relieve stress at the end of a long day, but they often say they feel stuck in a loop of endless content and design features that pull them in for longer. No parent judgment here—this is a case of tech design grabbing our exhausted attention and not letting go (see Tech Corner: The Designs That Drive Technoference section later in this chapter).

In experiments where parents used their smartphones in front of their infants, the parents who demonstrated heavier phone use habits also had more difficulty with repair, meaning that they struggled to reconnect with their infant and calm down together. Why might this be? If we get used to regularly smoothing away our parenting stress by turning toward our phone, we lose chances to practice the uncomfortable but worthwhile process of identifying and managing negative feelings.

On the flip side, when parents put phones away or turn off the TV during playtime, research shows that kids' play is more imaginative, parents find it easier to play along, and there is more talking back and forth—all things that support relationships.

What Contributes to Technoference?

Parent mental health challenges and emotional exhaustion: When I (Jenny) was a developmental behavioral pediatrics trainee, I met a mother and her 3-year-old son for a behavioral evaluation. The child was very stressed from being in a doctor's office and uncomfortable with his arm being squeezed with a blood pressure cuff. While I tried to engage this busy toddler, who wandered around the room and threw blocks, his mother looked at her phone for most of the visit. This mother's struggle to engage with her dysregulated child—and why she chose to avoid it through engaging with content on her phone—is totally understandable if we put ourselves in her shoes. Children with more sensation-seeking, intense emotions and big behaviors require a whole different set of parenting skills. Media is satisfying, frictionless, and tailored to our psychological needs, so interacting with it can often be more appealing than attending to a tantrumming child. Therefore, rather than dismissing her phone absorption as her being a "bad parent," over time we worked on behavior and relationship skill-building techniques and getting that child into preschool.

Practical Takeaway | **Supporting Parent-Child Relationships**

1. **What does the behavior mean?** First, during that visit we talked about what the child's difficult behavior was trying to communicate. All behavior is communication. Her child was using less mature forms of communication indicating "I'm overwhelmed" by throwing blocks. As part of my developmental testing, I found that he had a receptive and expressive language delay, so we were able to discuss the extra support he needed in expressing himself (starting with words like *help* or *I need a break*) and understanding instructions (eg, using a visual schedule to show what would happen next).
2. **What alternative activities can help manage the behavior?** We also discussed that he loves to throw things because his sensory profile is more sensation seeking. We planned out a few activities he could do at home to get this impulse out (ie, throwing balled-up socks into a laundry basket, running in a nearby park, and play wrestling) so that he didn't use it on other people.
3. **What therapies or supports are available?** I also referred him for speech and language therapy and occupational therapy to help with his delays. Getting him into low-cost preschool helped take some of the pressure off his mother to keep him occupied all day.
4. **Focusing on the relationship rather than just the media overuse.** This conversation revealed how much this mom loved her little ball of energy, but she felt ineffective in parenting him. Instead of judging her for using her phone, I focused on how she

could feel more connected with her son. I suggested that she take 20 minutes a day to play a game of his choice, with the phones away and TV off. This is an approach called **Special Time** that has been found to reduce oppositional behaviors in young children.

Feeling pressure to react and post: Social media has created a new set of expectations to maintain relationships online. In a 2026 study that my (Jenny) team conducted about social media designs, parents shared they resented the fact that some social media apps sent notifications telling them to come back to the app frequently, using fear of missing out (FOMO) tactics like telling them that they would miss a live stream, that someone they know had posted, or that someone had been looking at their profile. They also described pressure to perform their relationships on social media, such as wishing a family member a happy birthday publicly on social media even though they had already texted them their well-wishes.

Engagement-prolonging designs: Designs such as endless scroll and algorithms that predict what you might want to watch next have led many parents to indicate that they regretted staying up late consuming short-form videos on TikTok or Instagram, when they could have been sleeping. There's a tension between the "me time" that every parent deserves and the "wasted time" feeling of being stuck in a loop of content. The Tech Corner: The Designs That Drive Technoference section later in this chapter lists the main ways designs capture attention that could lead to technoference. In other words, don't blame yourself. Social media is designed to keep your attention on the platform's app.

Work demands: Sixty-plus-hour workweeks. Multiple jobs. After-hours emails and instant messages. Deadlines and expectations to be a "good worker" by showing that you are available all evening (even while getting the kids into the tub and then into pajamas). These expectations have expanded and exploded over the past 2 decades as the information economy started to dominate and more jobs involved sitting with a laptop. In the United States, Microsoft reported some pretty dramatic 2024 statistics showing how overworked adults are.

- Forty percent of people who are online at 6 am are reviewing email for the day's priorities.
- The average worker receives 117 emails and 153 Teams messages per day.
- Meetings after 8 pm have increased 16% year after year.
- Checking work emails on weekends is common.
- One in 3 employees reported that "the pace of work over the past 5 years has made it impossible to keep up."

In 2016, France even passed a right-to-disconnect law requiring that companies create an after-hours email policy with their employees to prevent the work-life overflow that many families experience.

In this book, we can't change the status of the economy or whether your boss expects you to answer emails after hours. But we can give you ideas of how to create the boundaries that you deserve—and the more these boundaries are normalized (or demanded) by parents, the easier it will be to enforce them.

Tech Corner | **The Designs That Drive Technoference**

Think about how often you see the following designs in a typical day:

Attention-capturing designs: When a parent needs something online, they are often flooded with pop-up discount offers, flashy thumbnail images, clickbait news items, or search recommendations that derail their train of thought (like when you put your cursor in the search bar and some scary trending search term like "when is the next pandemic" automatically pops up and you forget what you were searching for). All these design tricks extend time online and get parents to click, view ads, and generate data (which all = $$ to platforms), but they don't meet parent's goals of getting stuff done. If you don't like attention-grabbing designs, try to choose websites that don't rely on advertising (eg, use the National Weather Service website for weather information instead of ad-filled weather websites).

Designs that don't let you go: Infinite scroll (where you can see endless content with a flick of your thumb) and auto-playing videos are 2 classic examples of engagement-prolonging designs that lull users into lingering longer. Mobile video games also have endless levels that make it hard to disengage. Parents often regret that extra time they spent online. Helpful designs would let parents set an intention for how long they want to spend online and then nudge them off and let them go when the time is up. Until those designs exist, one solution is to set a timer when you start using an app with engagement-prolonging features. You can also set a time limit through the digital well-being/screen time features on your phone.

Data collection and psychological profiling: Data collection is invisible, so we don't often think about it, but it shapes the personalization that keeps us on social media and gaming platforms longer. Most platforms create *vectors* about us that signify our purchasing patterns and personality, which they share with companies called *data brokers* that sell the data to other companies. Kind of creepy. Some video game companies have even developed AI tools that help them predict just when a gamer is likely to disengage and then nudge that player with a prize or a treat to stay on longer. Some social media companies study our patterns of checking and send notifications just when they know they will be most successful in getting us to open the app. How can you resist this type of data profiling? You can reject cookies, delete your data from companies that allow this, use search engines that don't sell your data (like DuckDuckGo), or limit your time on social media and gaming platforms, which are the biggest offenders of data collection. This is a lot of work, so we really need data privacy legislation to make this easier. Tell your legislator.

Strategies to Reduce Technoference

Set Up Protected Times and Spaces for Parent-Child Connection

- Set up regular times when you feel connected with your family (even just once a day) and decide on times that technology will not invade. It helps to remember that a lot of technology platforms like social media, news, streaming video, and mobile games make more money the more you use them, so they have every interest in creating habits and being part of your regular downtime. But downtime with your children will pay off in terms of raising a well-adjusted human. Schedule daily playtime without technology. As we previously described, even 20 minutes per day of free play with your child can reduce negative and attention-seeking behavior.
- Look for routines that allow an opportunity to connect and check in with your teen. Before they are old enough to drive, you can turn taxi time into talking time as you take them to activities. Having tech-free time in the car is a great way to talk. Allow your child to choose the music in the car as long as they are willing to chat. If you have a pet that needs walking, take those walks together to embrace the time to catch up and factor in some physical activity as well.
- Create physical distance between you and the phone by placing it in a bag, bin, or box or on a shelf. You can use a focus setting or do-not-disturb feature that allows you to still receive urgent calls.
- Notice which apps take up the most of your time yet don't leave you feeling calmer and in control. This might be an app you doomscroll at night or one that makes you compare yourself with popular "momfluencers." You can look on your screen time settings to see which app you use for longest each day, identify the apps that drain your joy or attention, and try setting a time limit or uninstalling those apps for a while to see how it feels.

How communication can lead to connection

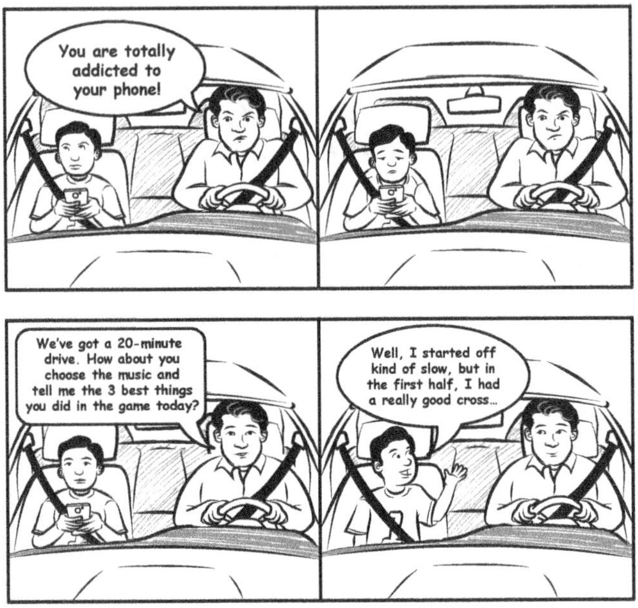
You are totally addicted to your phone!
We've got a 20-minute drive. How about you choose the music and tell me the 3 best things you did in the game today?
Well, I started off kind of slow, but in the first half, I had a really good cross...

Ask Your Kids About How Technoference Feels

- Kids (especially teens) are very observant and will likely notice when you or other adults are on tech often. If you are trying to set limits on *their* media use, yet *you* are scrolling away at night, they may call you out on this double standard. Ask them how it makes them feel when your attention is stuck on the phone.

Set Aside You Time

- Scrolling on a social media feed might seem like the easy way to relax at the end of a stressful day, but algorithms can always deliver a surprise of stress-inducing content. Instead, think of the offline activities that calm your mind and your body such as taking a walk, reading, making a cup of tea, or putting on music. By engaging in these non-digital activities, you're also role modeling healthy stress relief for your children.

Reel in Work Technoference

- Set expectations with your team or manager that you work only during work hours. If for some reason after-hours work is expected, communicate that there are times you won't be available, such as dinner and/or bedtime, and that you will check email afterward.
- Set away hours in Teams, Slack, or other work messaging platforms.
- Have an email signature that communicates your work hours.
- Leave your device in your workbag until the kids are asleep and then give yourself a set amount of time to manage your inbox, if need be.

Notice When Family Frustrations Are Driving Technoference

- When toddlers and preschoolers show negative behavior, such as big tantrums, hitting, and biting, it can make parents anxious or angry. Many parents say this makes them want to withdraw into their phone for some peace and quiet. But most young children don't know how to handle their emotions on their own. If a parent withdraws, the child might interpret this as rejection, and at the very least it will be a missed opportunity to help their child to learn coping strategies. Over time, this can lead to worse behavior in the child, who may escalate their behavior to get more attention from a withdrawn parent. Our advice is to first recognize when this withdrawal-into-the-phone habit is happening. Then, think of other ways to take a quick break (walking out of the room, taking deep breaths, texting a friend), self-regulate, refill your compassion tank, and then rejoin your child with a hug.
- Even if your child is not around, recognize whether your reaction to negative emotions is to automatically grab your phone. Reflect on whether you are often trying to escape emotional distress with distraction; if you are, try to come up with alternative emotional coping strategies. This could involve doing a brief meditation or breathing exercise, putting on music to sing or dance with, or talking to a friend. Teens tell us that journaling

and snuggling with a pet are also ways to relieve negative feelings without technology distractions.
- If you feel as if your teen is seeking their own "space" by being on their phone during family times, recognize this as a natural part of being a teen. You can set an expectation that they be phone- or laptop-free during family time but also allow them to find a safe space where they can be themselves without you there—this might be at another place like theater, music, sports, or school.

Practice Being Good Enough

- Repair is an important learning opportunity. If your child is an older teen and you make a mistake such as scrolling a bit too long and delaying getting dinner started, they will notice. Teens are very cognizant when adults mess up. Own your mistakes and make the mistake a moment to role model how to handle an error when this happens. Telling your child, "Whoa, I got a bit carried away with those cute cat videos; I better set an alarm next time," teaches them that it is OK to acknowledge an error and to seek ways to prevent it next time. It also shows them that you are OK with talking about the challenges of managing technology and makes it feel safe for them to talk to you if they have their own challenges.
- If you have a vacation or snow day where you all are stuck on your devices, don't beat yourself up. Talk with your kids about how it felt to be online all day. Easy? Exhausting? How does your body feel after all that time not moving or talking to each other? What do you feel like you missed out on?

Tech as a Connector

Some of the ideas in this section might seem obvious to you, but using tech as a connector often takes energy and planning for busy parents. The default in your household might be for everyone to be on their own device, so this section may help you intentionally set aside more shared and connected media use.

Alternatively, parents who generally are worried about screen time might be surprised to hear about the benefits of using media together with children, so it may open up new avenues for family connection that you hadn't thought of before.

Video chat. Some great examples of connections include FaceTime, Zoom, and Google Meet. (RIP Skype, which I [Jenny] used for video calls with distant family back in the day.) A 2021 study in the journal *Human Behavior and Emerging Technologies* surveyed parents and grandparents and found that families who used video chat for a regular check-in with loved ones had stronger feelings of closeness than those who used it infrequently. (It likely benefits grandparent mental health, too, but that hasn't been studied yet.) Babies can start video chatting more easily around age 15 to 18 months, when they have the cognitive and social skills to take turns and understand that the screen is showing someone they love in a different place. It can feel challenging to make a busy toddler or a bored teen focus on a video chat with loved ones. The following "Practical Takeaway: Tips for Connecting During Video Chats" box lists some creative ways to encourage this type of connection.

Practical Takeaway | **Tips for Connecting During Video Chats**

At any age, make video chats a consistent routine, such as talking with grandparents on Saturday mornings over breakfast. Make sure to turn off other tech that would compete for attention.

Younger Children

- Be animated, which can help keep younger kids stay engaged.
- Point to things on the screen to direct their attention.
- Give hugs and tickles on behalf of the person on the other side of the screen.
- Have the other person read, sing a song, or show things to the child.
- Have a puppet or the child's favorite stuffed animal come into the frame to interact with the other person.

Older Children and Teens

- Recall something cool that happened to your child or teen recently, such as a sports tryout or a chorus concert, that they may want to share with the other person.
- Make a routine of saving a joke that they heard recently to tell the other person.
- Critique pop culture events or recent movies or TV shows they have seen.
- Suggest that your teen ask grandparents, aunts, or uncles about what they were like as a teenager. What music did they like? What did they argue about with their parents? How did they meet their spouse?

Watching together. Parents can get the best snuggles from children (even teens, maybe) when watching a TV show or movie. Exhausted parents, we can't overstate the benefits of watching a movie or show that gives you ideas about how to talk to your children. Key titles in our parenting journeys include *Daniel Tiger's Neighborhood, Inside Out, Black-ish,* and *Love on the Spectrum.* These gems taught us how to talk about tricky topics: emotions, racism, living with disabilities, and dating. Even silly or shallow shows and movies connect us. Laughing together feels so good and creates inside jokes that can last for decades. You might be surprised by what your child learns, is scared of, or finds inspirational, and this gives you a peek into your child's mind.

Research shows that co-viewing is beneficial, but with certain caveats. Watching educational media with young children and repeating the concepts displayed in the show can build vocabulary, teach emotional coping skills (in the case of *Daniel Tiger's Neighborhood*), and help children comprehend what they saw and connect it to their everyday lives. However, as kids grow older, passively co-viewing can backfire. Picture this: You are watching a blockbuster movie that was just released to a streaming platform, and the main character is pretty violent, has a snarky attitude, and curses a lot. During commercial breaks, you see ads for mobile gambling apps. During this time, you say nothing. Studies have suggested that this type of passive co-viewing can be interpreted by teens as implicit approval of these activities.

As a result, you might see more snark, rude language, or interest in gambling from your teen. Therefore, in the teen years it's more important to be an active co-viewer. This includes role modeling a critical mindset about behaviors you don't approve of. This doesn't need to be a lecture: "I'm not crazy about the language that character uses. We can keep watching this movie as long as you agree to not use those words in school. Deal?" Also, talk about the themes that are important to you: "I like that the leading woman was strong; she wasn't just a pretty face" or "I feel like they didn't do a good job explaining how she got over her childhood losses."

Gaming together. Games can range from mindlessness to complex strategy and teamwork. Gaming as a team or competing with each other leads to focused time together, with a lot of laughing, maybe a little competitive banter, and great bonding. For my family (Megan), I started out trying to share old Gen X video game loves with my kids (think *Adventure* and *Pac-Man*). After tolerating my enthusiasm, they then looked for games that were a better fit. After a friend introduced them to the Nancy Drew games, it has become a family tradition to solve these mysteries together. While I would not win any awards for my in-game sleuthing and I cannot match up to Bess and George as a sidekick to help solve mysteries, I love the time together and the creative storytelling and puzzles.

Beyond the shared enjoyment, playing video games together allows parents to see how their child reacts to different game designs—either positively or negatively. Are they great at strategy? Maybe you can find good board games with similar strategies. Do they get upset a little when they aren't winning? (Tip—look for more collaborative games.) Are they fixated on collecting gems and in-game items, and perhaps this is why they keep begging you for money? This gives you insight into whether they are reward sensitive, which can contribute to more compulsive gaming. Tip—avoid the free games that involve pressure to make purchases (see Chapter 8). Also, skip the games that consist of guns and shooting. Experts in family gaming indicate that the easiest games for parents and kids to play together are racing games; sports games; and strategy games, especially where collaboration is key.

Texting. Adolescence is a time when teens are learning how to have complex conversations about heavy topics. These topics might include feelings such as being stressed, sad, worried, rejected, or irritated. I (Megan) remember when a 13-year-old patient was going through a tough time, and it really made it difficult for her to communicate with her dad. He couldn't

Practical Takeaway | **Co-Viewing Tips for Movie Nights**

Movie nights are a perfect opportunity for your family to zoom out from the small screen in your hands to the larger, easier-to-share screen in your living room. Schedule a movie on a regular night each week—most families choose Friday—and make a tradition of having your favorite food like pizza or snack like microwavable popcorn. If your kids argue about which movie to watch, rotate who gets to choose the movie each week. If they have a several-year split in their ages, Common Sense Media is a good source of recommendations for movies that will interest the whole family. If you have teens, make a list of Oscar-nominated movies that you want to see before the awards show.

Every once in a while, watch movies about technology and talk about digital literacy concepts.

- *Wreck It Ralph 2* uses humor to discuss the internet, scams, clickbait, and influencers.
- *Ready Player One* shows how greed in technology design can negatively influence people's online experiences. There are also interesting dystopian themes about how people want to spend all of their time in virtual reality (VR) because they feel that the real world is terrible.
- *The Matrix* raises existential questions about reality and AI.
- *Blade Runner* is a futuristic action movie that involves human-AI romantic relationships, which can spur conversations about AI consciousness and risks of being attached to AI.
- *Free Guy* talks about gaming design, ethics, and what different online gaming communities can look like.
- *2001: A Space Odyssey, War Games, Her, and Interstellar* all capture human relationships with AI (good, evil, and romantic).
- *The Social Dilemma* does a good job of explaining how online data can reveal a lot about our personalities and is used by marketers and algorithms to influence our behavior.

seem to say the right thing, and it made it difficult for her to feel comfortable expressing herself. It seemed as if every discussion would end up with the patient storming off to her room. Finally, 1 day after slamming the door, she texted her dad, "I'm sorry." And he texted back, "I'm sorry too." And so, a new phase began, when this parent-child relationship allowed for the use of texting when conversations got rough. Both the dad and the daughter knew that this phase would not last forever. At some point, the tough stuff would need to be talked out and not texted. But for that time, the use of text messaging was critical to keep them communicating.

The downside of parent-teen texting is that it can become what psychologist Sherry Turkle calls a *tether* that keeps you psychologically connected even when apart. For teens with anxiety or separation issues, it is especially important for them to experience handling life on their own, for example, getting through a stressful school day without needing to regularly check in with parents. For parents worried about their teen at school, because of bullying, fears of school shootings, or concern about the child's psychological state, it can be tempting to check in regularly to ensure that their child is doing OK. However, this unintentionally undermines the teen's sense of an autonomous, capable self (more about this in Chapter 11). School phone policies have made texting your teen less of an option in recent years, but our advice is to reflect on whether patterns of heavily texting your teen are placing you more in the "Micromanaging/Control" column of Table 1.1.

Research Corner | **Smartphone School Policy**

In a 2026 study, my colleagues and I (Megan) surveyed parents across the country to ask about school smartphone policies. We also asked parents about how often they contacted their child during the school day and whether their child had ever gotten in trouble for violating the school's smartphone policy. Twenty-five percent of parents reported contacting their child daily, and 38% shared that they contacted their child multiple times per day. This meant that more than half of parents contacted their child at school at least once every school day. We also found that parents who texted their child at school more frequently were more likely to have a child who had gotten in trouble for violating the school policy—another good reason to avoid texting kids during the school day.

Parent-Child Relationships: What If You Feel Disconnected Most of the Time?

Parent-child relationship problems can occur at any age. They usually appear as fussiness and discontent on both sides. We hear parents describing feelings such as they just don't know their child or being scared of the child's strong emotional reactions. When we ask what their child does well, or what activities make them feel most connected to their child, parents sometimes say, "Nothing." That is hard to hear because we want all parents and kids to see positivity in their relationship.

Parent-child relationship difficulties can also come with limited insight into the role that media is playing in disrupting family connections, maybe because it feels better when everyone's on their own device and there's no conflict.

We've noticed 2 common relationship dynamics around screens and technology.

- **Too much parental psychological control.** The parent feels anxious, ashamed, judged, or angry about their child's behavior. The child feels controlled and pushes back regularly with inappropriate language or aggressive behavior or shuts down and refuses to engage. The parent may put strict limits on the child's technology use, but the child sneaks or defies those limits. In this type of situation, a therapist is needed to help the parent feel comfortable using more autonomy-supportive (less controlling) parenting strategies, helping the child be more flexible, and doing regular relationship-building activities to increase trust and understanding.
- **The child is in control.** The parent might feel overwhelmed, burned out, or ineffective in managing their child's media use. The child is mostly determining when, where, and what media they use, even if it's problematic (ie, interfering with sleep, inappropriate content, or crowding out other healthy interests—see Chapter 14). In this case, a therapist can help with consistency in limit setting, putting settings on devices (eg, bedtime downtime settings), and problem-solving other activities that the child can do.

When we see families having difficulty connecting, we recommend starting small with one thing they feel will be an easy win—such as making a favorite recipe or watching a funny movie together—and prioritizing time for that daily when possible. A good therapist is incredibly helpful. They can get to know the child and their strengths and challenges and then work with families on practical ideas on how to make interactions more positive. This might include a different way to phrase things (eg, instead of "Come over here and listen to me," saying "I've got some things on my mind, and I want your input") or taking a beat before reacting to a child's attitude.

When children and teens don't feel understood at home, they often seek out places and people online that can relate. If they have a public social media account, are posting a lot, or seem desperate for attention, they can be easily targeted by child predators or manipulative ads for AI companions (see Chapters 3 and 4) or risky experiences (see Chapter 15). If they encounter negative experiences online, they might feel too ashamed to bring it to a parent they perceive as unsupportive. Therefore, work on parent-child relationships should always include communication strategies that are open, non-shaming, and consistent. Children need to know that they can come to a parent to talk about difficult things that happen offline or online.

Connecting the Dots

Parents are not perfect and don't need to pretend to be. If we can take stock of the different pressures we are feeling—from work to social pressure to judgment from others—we can get a clearer view of our relationship with technology and make it more balanced. We can increase the likelihood that tech is acting as a connector, rather than a disconnector, in our family.

- **Create an experiment:** Try some experiments at home in which you allow more interference from technology versus creating boundaries. What does it feel like to parent with your phone pinging for your attention versus putting it away for the evening? What does it feel like to engage in playtime with the TV on versus off? Talk with your kids about what felt different.

- **Talk to your friends:** Sharing effective tips with friends is one way to learn new digital boundaries. Ask them about how hard it is to get away from work or other online obligations. How do they set boundaries around email or work messages? How do they recognize when they are doomscrolling? How do they keep devices away from the dinner table? Crowdsourcing knowledge like this can help you realize how resourceful other parents are—and it allows you to commiserate about how difficult setting boundaries around technology can be.

Chapter 2

PEER RELATIONSHIPS

What we will cover

- How children and teens make friends
- How to support positive texting behaviors with friends
- How social media can amplify positive or negative peer relationships
- How to support positive peer relationships online
- How to prevent and respond to cyberbullying or other unwanted online contact

For some children, making friends comes easily. For other children—those with shyness, autism, attention-deficit/hyperactivity disorder (ADHD), mental health challenges, or a history of trauma—extra support is needed to make connections with other kids. This chapter will take you through the building blocks of friendships and how those relationships can be augmented or disrupted through digital media.

Why Making Friends Doesn't Come Easily to All Children

As a child, could you be dropped off at a new summer camp and have a new group of friends by the end of the day? Or were you the child who got a stomachache and felt overwhelmed with all the new faces, voices, and personalities? Did you like to jump right in, or did you need a few days to warm up to new people?

If you were in the second group, a shy child who needed more time to adapt to new social situations, you are part of the 15% to 20% of people with a more inhibited and slow-to-warm-up temperament. A lot of sensitive people were like this as children. Through watching other kids, positive experiences, and support from a warm teacher or counselor, children who are neurotypical but shy can develop a comfortable set of social skills that serve them well.

For many other children, such as those with autism or ADHD, lagging social skills may need more teaching or support. These include the following:

- **Social thinking:** This includes the ability to read various types of social cues ("Everyone's in circle time; I think I should sit down too") or see things from another's perspective ("My classmate's dog died, and she is feeling sad").
- **Social pragmatics:** This includes expressing the thoughts in your head and making sure they are being received by the other person.
- **Impulse control and self-regulation:** This involves staying calm and waiting for signals from another person before acting, not overreacting to something they say or jumping to conclusions.
- **Mental flexibility:** This involves the ability to stretch outside of your comfort zone and adapt to new social situations ("Hmm, everyone on the playground is playing tag, but I'm used to playing catch") rather than insisting everyone play your way.

These differences in social skills can translate to differences in peer relationships offline and online. Children with autism and ADHD may prefer the ease of online interactions in which they don't have to read facial expressions and can chat on an equal playing field with others. At the same time, children with underdeveloped social skills may be more susceptible to bullying or exploitation online because they overreact or over-trust other people. If your child struggles with social skills or making friends, our key message here is to support them in developing offline friends before they start searching for connections online. You can do this through the following:

- Ask their school to provide a social skills group or "lunch bunch" where they can practice playing games, having conversations, and being flexible with classmates.
- Find social skills opportunities outside of school, which could include social skills groups run by therapists but also clubs or sports in which your child can meet peers with shared interests such as LEGO, music, comics, theater, or particular games. Your neighborhood may also have opportunities for your child to connect with other kids such as on your block, in your apartment building, or through nearby locations such as YMCAs or libraries.
- Schedule a regular time to get together if there are family members your child connects with. This might be a weekly outing for pizza with an uncle or weekend get-togethers with cousins.

Peers and Media

Friendships in childhood often occur both around digital media and through digital media. Here are some examples.

- In early childhood, children might like watching popular movies together and then playing with or pretending to be characters from those movies such as cars, superheroes, or princesses.
- In the elementary school years, digital media can be a source of shared interests, such as popular movies or music or playing video games together. In my (Jenny) clinical work with children with autism, their amazing ability to remember facts often helps them connect with other children by talking about *Pokémon*, *Magic: The Gathering*, or all the different items in *Minecraft*.
- In the preteen and teen years, media becomes a crucial source of connection, especially for kids who are geographically or otherwise isolated (eg, kids in the hospital for chronic conditions such as cystic fibrosis or sickle cell disease).

Practical Takeaway | **Your Child's First Phone**

OK, the big question: When is your child ready for a phone? If you need to communicate with your child between households or to coordinate a tricky pickup schedule, then a flip phone may be appropriate for a child in elementary school through high school. This type of phone allows calling and texting, is relatively inexpensive, and is available through most carriers.

If you want to be able to track your child's location with GPS, a flip phone cannot do this—you would need a smartwatch-type device. The pros and cons of a smartwatch include the following:

- **Pros:** Typically, they are less expensive than a smartphone, kids can set alarms and reminders for chores, and parents can control who the child contacts and downtime settings.
- **Cons:** Kids can take them off and lose them, and they can come with distracting games.

A 2025 article in the journal *Pediatrics*, using data from the Adolescent Brain and Cognitive Development Study, found that children who received their first smartphone by age 12 had slightly higher rates of depression, sleep problems, and obesity than children who didn't receive a smartphone. Smartphones provide access to so many more things than children or teens need, so regardless of the age your child gets a first phone, make it simple and boring to start. This means you can get them a starter phone initially (there are several brands, such as Pinwheel, Gabb, and Bark, but just a warning that they all cost extra money) or you can use a traditional smartphone and lock it down. When getting a smartphone for a child or teen,

- Provide access only to the functions your child needs, usually phone, text, maps, and photos.
- Start with no games, social media, or browsers.
- Set up parental controls for content (blocking things like

pornography), contacts (to block scammers), downloads (so that you can oversee what they install), and in-app and online purchases.

- Set up downtime settings so that the phone can't be used at school or overnight (only for emergencies).
- Set time limits for the phone overall and for particular apps.
- Limit the data plan so that your child can use only certain apps when off Wi-Fi. I (Jenny) tried this with my older son, and it prevented him from getting into the habit of picking up his phone whenever he was bored while out and about in the community when Wi-Fi wasn't available.

Four Tips on Setting New Phone Expectations

1. Don't provide a full-octane smartphone; it provides too much access and can lead to distracting habits.
2. Don't have your teen expect that they can use it anytime of day or night. Create a set of guidelines or rules for phone use at home and consider making a Family Media Plan (a free tool created by the American Academy of Pediatrics [AAP]) offered on their parent-focused website HealthyChildren.org.
3. Set expectations that they should "pause for people" and look up from their smartphone when other people need their attention.
4. Set the expectation that you will talk about their relationship with their phone on a regular basis. If they are becoming too fixated on it, you will help them change things up to feel more balanced.

Texting: Figuring Out Social Rules and Boundaries

Texting and video chat are the best ways to have young teens stay connected with friends through media. Video chat is synchronous, so it allows children to respond immediately to what a friend says or have a live conversation. Texting is asynchronous, and kids can't see their friends' social cues, so it is a good learning opportunity on a few fronts.

Scenes from a first phone

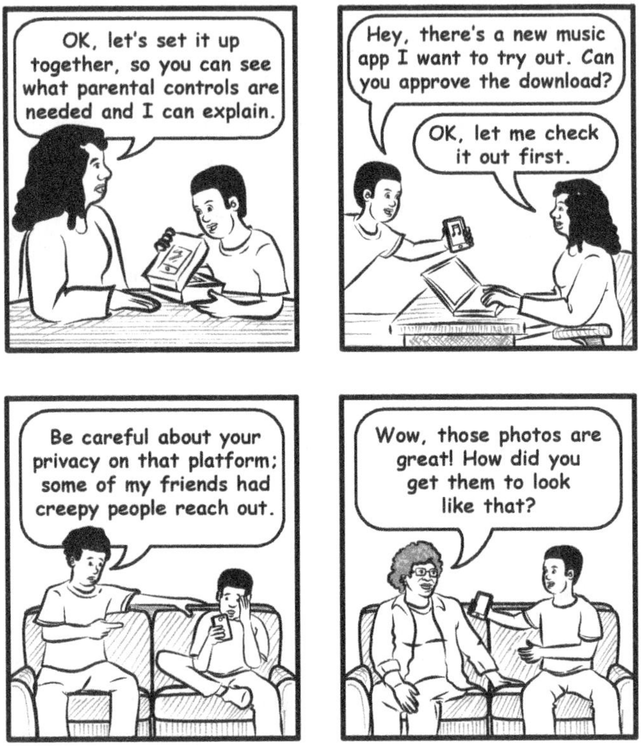

How much texting is enough, and how much is too much? At first, kids may want to share every thought or joke with friends, but this can be seen as spamming their friends. Reviewing your child's texts together, especially when they first are allowed a phone, can help you check whether they are sending a lot of texts without receiving a lot of replies.

Some Ways to Do This

- When your child gets a phone and starts to text, explain to them that this is a new way of communicating and that you want to support them in learning. To do so, sit together on a regular basis (could be 2 or 3 times a week to start, and gradually work to weekly check-ins). You can keep these relatively short and focus on listening to and learning from your child and helping them reflect on their thoughts. This will help reinforce positive and healthy ways to communicate. During that time together, the discussion can include the following:

  - Ask your child to pick a texting exchange that they feel really went well, and look at it together. Look for ways to compliment your child, maybe they did a thumbs-up when someone shared information to show support and acknowledgment, rather than changing the subject right away.
  - Ask your child to pick a texting exchange they are not sure about, and look at it together. Talk through the ways the words may have been interpreted and whether they would communicate differently next time. If it is relevant, bring up that when a texting string starts to go off the rails, it may be time for a phone call or just talking in person to avoid making things more confusing.

- Texts can be vague or lead to misunderstandings and hurt feelings. This is because kids use abbreviations, lingo, GIFs, emojis, or comments that are harder to interpret through a screen without the broader context or their friend's social cues or mannerisms. As with offline misunderstandings, be available to help your child unpack social difficulties they're experiencing online.
- What are their friends' phone boundaries? Some might have a lot of time away from their phone, and others may always respond right away. You can help your child recognize that all kids have different rules regarding their phone usage.

Some Ways to Incorporate Your Own Boundaries

- When you set limits on your child's phone communication, such as limiting access during family dinner, talk with your child about how they can communicate those rules to friends. Do they set a do-not-disturb message so friends know they are not able to respond? Does your child leave their phone in the other room during non-tech hours?
- Talk to your child about their friends' phone boundaries and what they think of those boundaries. Could some be incorporated into your family rules?

Research Corner | **What Teens Said Is the Best Age for a Phone**

One of my (Megan) favorite studies I have ever conducted is a study in which we asked tweens and teens what the right age was to get their own smartphone. You might think this was an opportunity for kids to say, "Whenever I want it!" However, in this research study, the 10- to 14-year-olds shared very nuanced thoughts about this question during focus groups. Their ideas boiled down to 3 key ideas: maturity, parental involvement, and accountability.

During discussions about the appropriate age for a smartphone, many tweens and teens were quick to dismiss the idea of an ideal age to get a smartphone. "I think it is not an age. I think it is more of a maturity thing," described one youth. Another participant stated, "I think it's more that you feel you're responsible enough to carry that burden." Youth described readiness skills as being mature enough to not lose the phone and to use it responsibly.

Tweens also described the importance of parents when a kid first receives a phone. They described that they expected, and hoped for, rules around when it was and was not appropriate to use the phone. They wanted rules that were specific and that parents would hold them to consistently.

One youth shared that they think smartphone rules should be clear and consistent: "I think that some rules are a little too subtle, like they aren't enforced as much as they should be. Some rules are a little less than what they should be, I think." Another youth described the importance of parental rules, stating, "I feel parents should have some degree of control over check[ing] your phone in at night. Or plug[ging] it in downstairs. They should definitely have rules in place about it. It shouldn't be something that you're kind of directing yourself on, having it free-for-all. Not at first anyways. Or for a long time."

Finally, tweens and teens described the importance of being held accountable for their actions when using the device. This included knowing how to treat others when communicating and avoiding harassing or cyberbullying. This also included avoiding problematic technology use. One tween shared, "I don't think there's like a specific age. But I think it's when they're responsible enough to not be addicted to it."

Some Ways to Navigate Texting Issues

- If your child talks to you about a text exchange gone awry, take a deep breath and sit down with them. Keep in mind you are there to provide support, not be a Monday-morning quarterback and tell them what they did wrong.
- Group chats or text threads are another way that preteens and teens solidify their friend groups and stay in regular touch about their daily lives. To some parents, this constant contact with friends may seem like too much, as many of us grew up with no texting and only phone calls with friends (on landlines). But to teens, the ability to bounce things off their friends and share lighthearted or stress-related moments feels meaningful and provides the support they value and need.

Definitions

GIF: GIF stands for *graphics interchange format*, which is a digital file that allows images to have both static/unmoving and moving/animated images. These are popular exchanges via text messages and show short, looping video clips used to express a reaction or express oneself.

Emoji: Emojis are pictograms, often a cartoon or comic-style picture, that people use to convey messages and emotional content. Popular emojis are faces expressing emotions, such as ☺ and ☹.

- Some group chats are large (think your teen's whole class) and can be full of drama or silliness. Talk to your child about how different group chats are feeling and that it's OK to mute the ones that are getting out of hand.

Research Corner | **The Meaning Behind Emojis**

Imagine this scenario: Your child is laughing and shows you a text from a friend that is an emoji of a hamburger. What does that mean? Is the friend eating a hamburger? Does it have some hidden meaning? How can you know? In a 2025 study, my colleagues and I (Megan) talked with older adolescents about the meaning of emojis in texting and how teens use emojis to express ideas and emotions. One key finding was that teens use emojis in texting to be funny and to stay connected, and this means that emojis don't always have a consistent or rational meaning.

One research participant described the following: "The sparkle [✨], or the pixie dust, I think was originally used to like enhance the meaning of something, or like making it aesthetic in some way. But now I'm just using it for random words that it doesn't really make sense in—but it's like funny in a way (laughs). It's kind of like ironically."

Another participant described that "there was like the chair emoji [🪑], which like people would just use it to be funny and like the point of it was that it had no meaning."

During adolescence, teens are developing shared bonds with friends. For some teens, having nonsense emojis in texting to represent a shared joke or just be funny is an essential part of that experience.

Chatting Through Video Games

Chatting doesn't only happen through text. In many online video games or virtual reality, there is a social component. Many parents we have talked to didn't realize this about games like Roblox or Fortnite before their child started playing them, so they didn't realize they needed to set up house rules and privacy settings. Here are some rules to consider.

- Turn off the in-game chat or only allow chatting with kids your child knows in real life. Teach them that untrustworthy adults have been known to pretend they are kids in online games (they may know this if they have heard adult voices in games). One patient told me (Jenny), "I always know it's an adult if they can type really fast." Other patients have incorrectly assumed, "Oh no, there are no adults playing Roblox—it's a kids' game." Don't assume that your kids know to be safe; talk about not chatting with strangers or sharing personal information and always keeping their chats private.

- Make an effort to occasionally be nearby and listen in during games where your child voice chats with friends. Placing the gaming console in a shared space in your home, like a living room or TV room rather than a bedroom, can make this easier. Monitoring the gaming banter will give you insight about whether your child is having mostly positive or age-appropriate interactions online (eg, teasing, competitive trash-talking) or whether you feel it is veering into abusive or inappropriate language.
- Set limits about language. In my (Jenny) experience with boys with ADHD, many become disinhibited and can push limits while chatting online. I recommend that parents set limits about what is considered OK language to use, such as no cursing or slurs, but mild rude humor might be OK to some parents. If the child or teen can't adhere to these expectations, then the chat gets turned off or they take a break from that particular game.

Social Media: How Tech Designs Shape Online Friendships

In addition to texting and video chat, teens do a lot of friendship building, maintenance, and communication through social media platforms such as Snapchat, Instagram, TikTok, or Discord. Many of the positives and negatives of friendships on social media are amplified by design features that are important for parents to understand.

Being Supported and Understood

The most revolutionary thing about the invention of the internet was connecting people around the world who share interests and otherwise couldn't have met in person. Fandoms and chat rooms popped up around books, video games, fashion, you name it. These were usually smaller groups, sometimes run by a moderator to make sure members were respecting each other. With the advent of Facebook in 2004, affinity groups expanded to

Practical Takeaway | **"My Child/Tween Is Begging for Social Media. What Do I Do?"**

Studies show that kids who start a social media account around 8 to 12 years of age have more problems than those who waited until they were older to start using social media. In a 2022 study from the journal *Computers in Human Behavior,* author Linda Charmaraman and colleagues found that children 10 years and younger and tweens ages 11 and 12 who started an underage account had higher rates of problematic (compulsive) usage, more fear of missing out (FOMO), and less empathetic behavior online. Developmentally, it may be that children and tweens have weaker judgment and less self-control and overfocus on likes and friend counts. This same research group found in a 2021 study that about 20% of 11- to 14-year-olds reported body dissatisfaction due to social media, which was primarily reported by girls. Reasons included not being thin enough, not being attractive enough, and disliking their body shape. For these reasons, we don't recommend social media use before age 13. Some governments are now mandating a minimum age of 16.

If your child wants social media earlier than the minimum legal age, we advise that you stick within the platform age limits. Encourage other ways to engage with peers, either online through supervised gaming or texting or offline by finding a club, theater or music group, or sport that provides regular friend contact.

Some ways to talk about this with your child are to consider including comparisons with other age-based limitations, such as getting a driver's license at age 16 or voting at age 18. It can be helpful to frame this discussion around the fact that there are not huge numbers of age-based rules in our society but that when those exist, they are typically tied to protection, and we want to respect that. If you as a parent allow access to social media and allow your child to lie about their age online, this could set an unhelpful precedent that this is an OK approach in handling other things such as driving, voting, or drinking.

tens of thousands of members, and groups were recommended to users who were profiled to have similar interests. Although social media can help people discover others with similar interests, it also can create echo chambers, online communities where everyone has the same values, which has been thought to contribute to political polarization. Unfortunately, the same automated algorithms that can connect old high school friends can also connect groups of people with the same nefarious interests, such as child sexual abuse/exploitation.

So, while the nature of online groups has shifted as the designs of internet platforms have evolved, it's important to realize that a main motivation for teens to use social media is to find "their people." Some examples we have heard from our patients include the following:

- A subreddit about their favorite video game where other "nerds" share tips and insights
- A TikTok community where members share their anime drawings and seek feedback
- A suicide recovery community where members support each other in their recovery journeys
- A lesbian, gay, bisexual, transgender, queer (or questioning), asexual (or allied), intersex (LGBTQAI+) community where members share their negative and positive stories about coming out and understanding and embracing their identity

Think of how good it feels to walk into a room, find your best friends, share inside jokes, and feel a sense of being valued. When children don't experience this feeling offline, they often seek it online. If your teen seems to be socializing more online than offline, then talk with open-minded curiosity about their online friends and how they treat each other and think about other offline communities where they might find belonging as well. For children who aren't naturally fitting into one of the usual offline groups (eg, sports or school clubs), other alternatives might include music, theater (especially an inclusive and noncompetitive theater group), a book club if they enjoy reading, a crafting group, or an organization that aligns with their interests and has volunteer opportunities (eg, an animal shelter for animal lovers or a food bank for kids who like to cook).

When Friendships Became Quantified

Social media has designs that can both support friendships and make users feel insecure. Myspace and Facebook were some of the first platforms that commodified the concept of "adding a friend" into a quantifiable unit. They knew that the more friends a user had, the longer they stayed on the platform, so it became a central part of the Facebook experience to be able to count the number of friends you accumulated through recommendations. Similarly, Snapchat quantified the closeness of different friends with Snap Streaks, the count of how many days in a row you shared Snap messages or photos with a friend.

Younger teens can overfocus on these visible counts of friendship and popularity. School-age kids and young teens are more concrete thinkers, which means they take things at face value and don't yet think about concepts like friendships in abstract, less measurable terms. Interviews of children and teens by the UK group 5Rights Foundation in 2023 explored how they think about friend counts and likes. Socially anxious teens reported that quantifying relationships increased their anxiety. One 16-year-old stated, "It becomes almost stressful to post anything because the amount of likes you get is your social standing. Your popularity or how much you're liked is based upon numbers on a screen." Rather than focusing on the *quality* of their developing relationships, many teens

Practical Takeaway | **Settings and Controls**

As a parent, you can support your child by helping them not create a social media account too young (see "Practical Takeaway: When Are Teens Ready for Social Media?" box later in this chapter), not overfocus on the quantity of friendships and instead focus on the quality of the friendships they have, and turn off public friend/follower counts through the platform's settings page if available. For some app-based or video games like Roblox, you can set parental controls so that you must approve your child's in-game friends. Talk to your child about only accepting friend requests from people they know in real life.

overfocused on the *quantity* of approval from online contacts. As a 13-year-old stated, "[There is the] pressure of losing your friends and ending life-long friendships if you forget to send a Streak one day."

Performing Friendships in Public

Teens enjoy posting about and tagging each other in photos as a way to share the fun of being on social media. This can amplify the feelings of connections friends feel for each other, but it can also make other teens (especially those not included in the post) feel left out. Teens say there are many tech designs that contribute to FOMO and the social comparison that they feel when they see peers having fun online. These features include photo tagging, like counts on photos or posted stories, designs that symbolize the strength of a relationship (eg, Snap Streak counts), or online status indicators (eg, seeing a green dot next to their friend's avatar, indicating they are online, but not getting any response from that person). Parents should be aware that there are several features that raise the social stakes for teens online and that can make them feel more or less included in their peer group.

If your teen is going through a tough time with peers, including being bullied or left out, this might also be amplified online. They might need more breaks from social media or video games to avoid this stress while they work on connecting with peers offline.

Experiencing social missteps is a typical part of navigating peer relationships in middle school and high school. Children don't always realize they are being inappropriate or showing off. The best way to learn from these types of social missteps is to get calm, constructive feedback that helps them learn what went wrong and how to repair the situation. Guess what type of feedback is rarely calm and constructive? Social media comments. People tend to be more single-minded and even vitriolic in their social media responses when they disagree with others (you've probably seen this in your own social media feed), which can worsen the situation for teens by making them feel "canceled" or wanting to double down on what they said. Encourage your teen to come to you with social media drama if they need help unpacking why they received a negative reaction from peers. We also encourage that your teen's social media account be private—so that they are only sharing posts with their in-group—which prevents people they don't know from accessing their account.

Practical Takeaway | **When Are Teens Ready for Social Media?**

There are public debates about the best age for starting social media accounts. In Australia, the age was increased to 16 in 2025, which was both praised and criticized. The truth is that research shows older teens, young adults, and adults can all struggle with problematic social media use. But developmentally, teens do become more mature as they get older. Therefore, if your child turns 13 and is not interested in or ready for social media, follow their lead. Not every child needs social media. There are other ways to engage online or in person, and there is no known benefit of encouraging your child to interact with social media if they don't want to.

If your child is 13 and wants social media access, what do you do? Most youth want to start with a particular platform, and it is usually the platform where their friends are. (This is better than opening multiple social media accounts on different platforms, which will be harder for you to monitor.) Take a little time to learn about that platform on your own. One good resource for this is the Common Sense Media Parents' Ultimate Guides to different social media platforms. Our AAP Center of Excellence on Social Media and Youth Mental Health also has an online glossary that outlines all the safety and parent supervision settings available on different social media sites.

Ideally, sit with your child together and look through the settings and get a general sense of the social media content they are seeing. Do your best to ask open-ended questions: "What do you think about this?" or "Tell me about your friend who is commenting a lot." This sets up the expectation that you can look at their platform together and that you will ask questions and listen to their thoughts. Over time, if using the platform seems to be affecting them negatively, you can talk about taking a break from it.

If you, as a parent, don't use social media and have strong feelings about its effects on politics, misinformation, or societal polarization, that's OK. Share these concerns with your teen. See if they have heard about them or have the same opinions—and why or why not. You can role model a critical thinking mindset and can help them be intentional about when and why they want to start a social media account.

As your child eventually joins other social media platforms, it's a good idea to continue this type of regular communication practice. It shows your teen that it's important to be mindful of what social media platforms they engage with, as some carry higher risks of negative social comparison, misinformation, or harassment. Social media companies are not a monolith; some appear to be working hard to have safer experiences for teens, while other "digital well-being" initiatives might be window dressing. Take time once in a while to ask them to show you content on the social media platform they are using the most—maybe content that is funny (cute cat videos) or meaningful to them (homecoming pics) or worrisome to them (video of 2 people fighting). Ask questions, listen, and repeat.

Anonymity and Online-Only Friendships

Online-only friendships have increased since the COVID-19 pandemic. In 2021, the Survey Center on American Life found that 39% of US adults had friends who they only interacted with online. Rates of online-only friendships were similar (38%) in a US survey of 10- to 14-year-olds published in the *Journal of Clinical Child & Adolescent Psychology* in 2022, with significantly higher rates (46%) in teens experiencing suicidal ideation. Sometimes the only thing your teen might know about an online "friend" is their username and how they act in a video game or chats. Anonymity allows people to open up more and speak their mind online, which helps when discussing stigmatizing topics like suicide. But it also can increase the risk of deception and bullying because people's actions are separate from their offline identity. For example, therapists we have talked to described their patients being pressured into doing things by online acquaintances—in one case, a child with autism felt pressured to draw and share nude anime pictures that they later felt ashamed of.

How to Support Your Children in Positive Online Relationships

Think of online peer relationships as an extension of your kids' offline peer relationships. The same social skills you would want them to demonstrate in school, on their sports team, or while hanging out at a friend's house apply to how they should act in social spaces online. If they wouldn't mock someone to their face, they shouldn't do it on any social media app, platform, or video game. If you think a little competitive banter is OK on the soccer field, then keep the same limits around chatting during video games.

- Talk about children's online interactions regularly so that they see this as a normal part of checking in with you. This is especially important before starting a new account or getting a new device. Use curious conversational tactics (see Conversation Tips: Peer

Research Corner | **Friend Requests**

In one of my (Jenny) studies about the game Roblox, I interviewed kids ages 8 to 14 about how they navigated friend requests from other players. Many kids said they accepted friend requests from anyone who "seemed nice"—they had no idea that adults might be posing as kids on the game. One participant described being followed by another player who wanted to "online date" them and wouldn't leave them alone. They weren't sure how to get this person to leave them alone, and they thought it was their fault, so they didn't share it with their parents. As a research team, we felt an ethical obligation to tell their parents, who appreciated the advice on setting up privacy controls and how to talk with their child about it.

Unfortunately, many kids may not realize that there are inappropriate people on video games and social media, which could lead to chatting with someone who is dangerous. The good news is that rules and expectations work. Other kids in this study shared that their parents implemented clear rules about who they could friend online, so they only accepted friend requests from or chatted with people they knew in real life, such as their neighbors or cousins.

Relationships section later in this chapter) so that your child doesn't feel the impulse to shut down, minimize, or lie. If they know you've got their back, but you won't overreact, they will be more likely to come to you and be honest.

- Normalize time away from technology. Teens are going to feel pulled to their friends through texting and social media, which can build the false expectation that all messages should be responded to immediately. Healthy relationships have boundaries, including not being near the phone at night or sometimes turning off notifications to focus on other activities such as taking a walk or completing homework.
- Help your child develop online social skills—especially perspective taking—such as discussing how their posts or texts affect other people or understanding how other people might be offended by a post your child thinks is funny.

Practical Takeaway | **Safety Features**

If your child or teen uses platforms or games that allow anonymity or avatars, such as Reddit or Roblox, you can use a few safety features to help keep online connections safe.

- Use parental control settings, if available, so that you have to approve your child's online friends.
- Talk to your child about who they chat with online and how those people behave, and let them know there can be inappropriate adults in kids' games.
- Help kids recognize what healthy online interactions look and feel like. They should generally be supportive, fun, and nonthreatening. If they get an uncomfortable feeling about people online, they should trust their gut and not interact with them.
- Let them know about mental health resources such as seeking out a therapist, the 988 hotline, The Jed Foundation, and The Trevor Project if you think they are seeking out online relationships to talk about mental health symptoms.

- Pay attention to overall social dynamics in your child's friend group. If they are talking about being enemies with anyone, being in a fight, or feeling like others are mean, explore how much this is happening in person versus online. Your child's behavior or social missteps might be part of the negativity, so think together about healthier ways to handle conflict.
- Keep your teen's accounts private so that random trolls and strangers can't harass them.
- Encourage offline community. Everyone needs a strong offline community to feel a sense of belonging and being cared for. If this isn't happening in school, talk with teachers, administrators, or the school social worker about how your child is struggling and what could help. Talk with your teen about where they can find their people—and be ready that it might mean an awkward first step such as trying out for a play or meeting new people at a comic bookstore.

Conversation Tips | **Peer Relationships**

"Who do you hang out with on that game? Do you chat with anyone?"

"How can you tell who is a kid and who is a grown-up? Do you think people lie about their identities online?"

"What do you do if you see players stalking or bothering friends online? How do you handle that?"

"How do you handle it when people are mean online?"

One approach we learned from a therapist involves drawing out friendship circles on a piece of paper. In the closest circle (the bull's-eye), teens can put the names of the friends they trust the most or who they would go to in an emergency. On the next outer circle, they list people they like and consider to be friends at school or elsewhere but who are not their best friends. On the next outer circle, they list a few classmates or acquaintances. For kids they argue with or they don't get along with, help them figure out whether to put them farther out or not in a circle at all. Now, what about people they know online? Which circle would they go in? Help them compare the experiences of friends they know offline and those they know only online.

Bullying and Online Harassment

Cyberbullying is defined as a repeated activity conducted by using digital technologies that is intended to hurt, intimidate, or ridicule another person. In 2023, the Youth Risk Behavior Surveillance System found that 16% of high school students reported being cyberbullied, and rates were closer to 20% to 30% in middle school students. Being a person who is bullied or a bully is linked with mental health problems, school failure, and suicidal thoughts.

Cyberbullying is not uncommon, and it feels terrible. If you think about the fact that preteens and teens are highly sensitive to social feedback from their peers, you can imagine how upsetting it feels to be rejected, disliked, and ridiculed—whether this is public (done over social media or group chat, so others can see) or private (done through private chat, sometimes anonymously). In 2022, the Pew Research Center reported that more than half of teens surveyed indicated that they've been called names or put down online, and this negatively affected their sense of self-worth.

Being bullied feels shameful, so kids often don't want to talk about it. Our biggest message for parents is this: If you create the space for kids to come to you about negative experiences online, you'll be much more likely to detect bullying and help support your child. In a study my colleagues and I (Megan) did, we interviewed parents and teens separately and asked about experiences with cyberbullying. Somewhat surprising to us was that about 10% of teens reported bullying and their parents reported that their child had experienced none. Another 10% of parents reported that their child had been bullied but the child did not report any bullying experiences. This study clearly highlighted how important it is for youth and parents to be on the same page in understanding the experiences the youth has had so that parents can provide support. Conversations are key to getting on the same page.

What Is Cyberbullying?

Online bullying can take many forms. It can include the following:

- Harassment (insults, calling names, making degrading comments or threats)
- Spreading lies or rumors

- Posting embarrassing photos or videos
- Impersonating another person
- Outing another person (eg, as LGBTQAI+ or another aspect of their identity they may be keeping private or posting their address or contact information publicly)
- Trickery (gaining an individual's trust and then using online media to distribute their secrets)
- Exclusion (excluding an individual from activities)

What we know from research is that cyberbullying can typically lead to offline bullying as well, also called *face-to-face bullying*. Bullying is more common toward LGBTQAI+ youth, neurodivergent youth, youth of color,

Research Corner | **Bullying Versus Cyberbullying**

There is a "uniform definition of bullying" that was put forward by the Centers for Disease Control and Prevention (CDC) and US Department of Education in 2014 to describe bullying and cyberbullying. It states, "Bullying is any unwanted aggressive behavior(s) by another youth or group of youths who are not siblings or current dating partners that involves an observed or perceived power imbalance and is repeated multiple times or is highly likely to be repeated. Bullying may inflict harm or distress on the targeted youth including physical, psychological, social, or educational harm."

In a 2018 study, my colleagues and I (Megan) asked youth and parents to share examples of cases and descriptions of cyberbullying to see how well they matched up to that CDC definition. Our participants created a highly varied selection of example cases and descriptions of cyberbullying. Some cases included terms that were closely tied to cyberbullying experiences, such as "flaming" and "online harassment." However, no single described case included all components of the bullying definition. This study shows that while a definition of bullying is helpful, an individual's experience with bullying does not have to exactly meet all parts of the definition to be a negative and potentially harmful experience.

and youth who have overweight or are living in larger bodies. A 2018 study of risks showed that 84.6% of LGBTQ+ students reported being verbally harassed, 65% heard homophobic remarks, and 40.1% reported being physically assaulted at school in the past year because of their perceived (or assumed) nonheterosexual sexual orientation. A 2018 meta-analysis combined data from multiple studies to make a much larger and more powerful study, and it showed that youth who had overweight had approximately 20% increased odds and youth with obesity had 50% increased odds of experiencing bullying compared with their peers of average weight. Some bullies crave power, so they single out individuals they see as having less power or "social capital" and make them feel smaller so that they can seem stronger.

Possible Signs of Cyberbullying

As we previously noted, kids may not feel comfortable talking about cyberbullying or might not even understand that rude interactions with their classmates or frenemies are bullying. A parent might notice these social challenges if they see their child being more stressed or nervous whether on their devices or not. They might seem more secretive or irritable and not want to talk about their day. The stress created from bullying can lead to children avoiding school, having trouble sleeping, or seeming more withdrawn. Signs of depression include not enjoying activities they usually participate in, having trouble focusing and making decisions, negative outlook or negative self-talk, or thoughts about harming themselves or others.

If you see these types of shifts in your child, it's time to try a few things to see if they will open up.

- Use open-ended questions (see Conversation Tips: Peer Relationships section earlier in this chapter).
- Try involving another family member, another trusted adult, their therapist (if they have one), or their pediatrician, if they still won't respond.
- Talk about what types of limits they want to put on their device use to make time for other positive activities, including talking to you.
- Try taking walks or drives or watching movies together to create a calmer space for difficult conversations.

Research Corner | **Managing Cyberbullying**

There are a few aspects of cyberbullying that can make it complicated to manage. One is that there can be an overlap between "traditional" bullying and cyberbullying. In a 2018 study, my colleague and I (Megan) created focus groups with both parents and teens to ask about perspectives and experiences with cyberbullying. One teen noted that cyberbullying by someone you know is harder to deal with than cyberbullying by someone you don't know or someone who remains anonymous.

> *"I feel like combating cyberbullying when it's coming from someone you don't know is much easier 'cause you can just turn it off, you can block them or something, but when it's cyberbullying from someone you know, probably someone at school, you can't just turn them off because you've got to see them the next day."*

This idea of cyberbullying being harder to deal with when it comes from someone you know was expressed in multiple teen focus groups. They also expressed that when cyberbullying occurs with someone you know, the victim often experiences cyberbullying from the perpetrator at home and traditional bullying from the perpetrator at school.

Stopbullying.gov Recommendations

If your child or teen is experiencing cyberbullying, check out resources from StopBullying.gov, which include steps such as the following:

- Don't respond to and don't forward cyberbullying messages.
- Keep evidence of cyberbullying. Record the dates, times, and descriptions of instances when cyberbullying has occurred. Save and print screenshots, emails, and text messages. Use this evidence to report cyberbullying to web and cell phone service providers and social media sites.

- Block the person who is cyberbullying, and report the bullying to the online platform.
- Report to law enforcement if the bullying includes the following:
  - Threats of violence
  - Child sexual abuse/exploitation or sending sexually explicit images or messages
  - Taking a photo or video of someone where they would expect privacy
  - Stalking and hate crimes

Help your child or teen take breaks from technology and reconnect more with the activities and people that give them joy and meaning. A therapist can be helpful to process your child's feelings, but don't underestimate the role you play in talking things through and problem-solving.

Connecting the Dots

Children and teens are naturally driven to connect with peers and enjoy the positive feedback they get from friends. As they grow older, more of this will happen online, and whether these experiences are positive or negative are shaped by your kid's peer group, the designs of the platforms they use, and the oversight you provide. Here are a few things you can do to explore these ideas more with your family.

- **Try a family experiment:** When your child receives a device or a gaming/social media account, talk about their new online interactions with their peers: When they interact online, what feels different than offline? What's missing, and what's better?
- **Talk to your friends:** Ask about texting and social media boundaries. When are the kids not available to each other, and when are the full-access times? This might help kids feel less FOMO when they have to turn the gaming console off or put their phone away before bed.

Chapter 3

PARASOCIAL RELATIONSHIPS

What we will cover

- What parasocial relationships are and why they matter
- Leveraging young kids' relationships with media characters
- Influencer effects on kids and teens (and even parents!)
- Parasocial relationships with AI chatbots
- Supporting kids' critical thinking about influencers and AI

Think about a character you loved in early childhood. Depending on when you were born, it might be Oscar the Grouch, Snoopy, Elmo, Bob the Builder, a fuzzy beast from *Yo Gabba Gabba!*, or Minnie Mouse. Did you have stuffed animals of this character that you carried around with you? When you think back, do you get a nostalgic and warm feeling about them?

Now think about a pop star, actor, or athlete you admired back when you were a teen. Did you have a poster of them up on your bedroom wall? Did you try to copy any of their dancing styles, hairdos, or sports moves?

Why do we connect emotionally with characters or celebrities, even though we don't know them in person? These parasocial relationships with media characters are common throughout childhood and into adulthood—and, as we review in this chapter, they can be used positively or used for manipulation.

Definition

A **parasocial relationship** is an imagined, one-sided connection in which a person develops a strong sense that they know and have a bond with a media figure, such as a fictional character, an influencer, or a celebrity. These feelings of intimacy and familiarity exist only on the side of the individual, who experiences a bond despite the lack of reciprocity.

Magical Thinking and Parasocial Relationships

Young children are magical thinkers, which means that they explore and explain life circumstances with creative, out-of-the-box explanations and stories that don't always align with reality. They are not logical thinkers yet, so they let their imagination fill in the blanks of the unknowns in the world. They may think that monsters under the bed are real, worry about getting sucked down the tub drain, or believe that fairies deliver money in exchange for teeth. I (Jenny) remember, as a young child, worrying that a grapefruit tree would grow in my stomach if I accidentally swallowed a seed at breakfast!

Magical thinking is an essential stage of cognitive development because it helps children make sense of the world, process emotions, and become flexible problem-solvers. It also shapes who (or what) children attach to: We've known children who name their family's car, feed their stuffed animals, or think their Alexa speaker is alive. Our minds naturally project humanlike qualities onto nonhuman things, called *anthropomorphizing*, and this is most pronounced in early childhood.

The Upside

An interesting aspect of parasocial relationships is that young children learn much more effectively from beloved media characters. A 2011 study published in *Media Psychology* compared how 2-year-olds in the United States learned the new skill of stacking cups from Elmo with how they learned it from a puppet equally beloved in Taiwan, but unknown to US toddlers, named DoDo. Toddlers paid more attention to, and learned much better, from Elmo—even though DoDo said the exact same words. Research shows that young children trust, learn, and absorb role modeling from characters they've developed an attachment to.

When you see a beloved character doing a behavior you'd like to see more of in your child (oh, where to start...cleaning up toys? taking turns? brushing their teeth?), point it out. Make sure that episode winds up on repeat a few more times. Your child may be more likely to try something because they witnessed Bluey doing it.

Sometimes the benefits of parasocial relationships are brief and simple. I (Jenny) recall my older son having a great memory for what happened in shows such as *Thomas & Friends* and using it as a script for what he felt in everyday life. He would bring out Sir Topham Hatt quotes such as "This is causing confusion and delay!" when life got too busy, and I would occasionally tease him about being a "bossy boiler" when he was being inflexible. My (Megan) kids would use the Sir Topham Hatt classic "My doctor has forbidden me to push!" when trying to avoid doing a chore. Sometimes TV characters give us words that we otherwise wouldn't have chosen to explain a situation but that really resonate with our kids.

The Downside

There may be characters your child has developed a parasocial relationship with that are mean, greedy, or manipulative. My (Jenny) research lab watches a lot of YouTube to understand the media exposures to toddlers in our studies. We collect the links of YouTube videos they watch so that we can evaluate how educational, positive, or commercialized the video content is. This also gives us insight into what the algorithm is recommending to little ones.

During this research, we noticed a phenomenon we call *wish fulfillment* that happens a lot more on YouTube than on traditional TV or videos. Kid influencers make videos where a camera follows them around while they do things many kids wish they could do on a regular basis—eat cake and candy bars, unbox and play with popular toys, or dress up like Disney princesses. They (or whoever produces the video) realized that these high-pleasure experiences attract a lot of clicks from kids, who have less impulse control and whose attention is more easily drawn to shiny things. These influencers often role model overconsumption or overfocus on appearance and sometimes play pranks on parents or sneak sweets behind a parent's back. Because of parasocial relationships, children could easily be influenced by these videos to want the same sweets or toys or to copy rude behavior.

Like we talk about more in Chapter 8, it's important for parents to recognize that online recommender feeds often feature exciting, attention-capturing content over the type of content you'd rather your child watch, such as kind or wise role modeling from characters. They may use "clickbait" to get your child to follow links (see the following definition). The solution is to watch along, identify the influencers or characters you don't care for, teach your kids why that behavior doesn't align with your values, and block those channels or choose another platform.

Definition

Clickbait is a tactic used by online creators to grab attention, usually through a headline or thumbnail illustration that encourages the user to click to engage with that piece of content. In other words, it "baits" people through their curiosity, emotions, or biases and can often be misleading or deceptive. Children might be more susceptible to clickbait because of their underdeveloped critical thinking skills and higher curiosity.

Encouraging In-App Purchases

YouTube isn't the only platform where my (Jenny) research assistants spend hours and hours of time. We also study the apps that children use on their tablets and smartphones. In Chapter 8, we will talk more about the learning potential from apps, but let's take some time in this chapter to focus on the undesired behaviors of some of the characters in those apps.

Research Corner | **Advertising in Apps**

One of my (Jenny) studies, published in 2018, looked at how advertising shows up in kids' apps. We downloaded and played hundreds of apps, recording when ads appeared, what those ads were for (surprisingly some about bipolar disorder treatment, wine distributors, and a video game where Santa shoots everyone), and other ways the app tried to make money off of gameplay. In several apps, a character even encouraged the child to make in-app purchases.

- In one beloved doll's fashion app, the character commented about how much she liked the sparkly shoes; these shoes were locked, and a purchase was required if the child wanted to give them to the doll.
- In a dentist app, a character cried when the player didn't make an in-app purchase to buy items like a drill that worked faster.
- In another beloved doll's bakery app, the characters order cakes that the player must make with certain ingredients. During the first few attempts, all the ingredients were free. You baked the cake, you gave it to the character and her friends, and they praised you. Then, ingredients were locked. If you only used free items and didn't buy the ingredients that the characters said they wanted in their cake, they replied, "Oh, that's OK. You can eat it," in a disappointed voice.

These are examples of manipulative parasocial relationships. When the study came out, the Federal Trade Commission was notified, and even a senator wrote a letter complaining that these unfair practices in children's apps needed to be stopped. Unfortunately, nothing came of it, so it remains on parents' shoulders to be aware: This type of purchase pressure can and does still occur in kids' apps. To avoid it, parents can avoid free apps; paid apps and those requiring subscriptions don't usually have this type of purchase pressure. App reviews are also available on Common Sense Media's website.

Teen Development and Parasocial Relationships

As we talk about in Chapter 11, identity development happens throughout childhood and into adulthood. But adolescence is a key period of identity development, dominated by questions such as *Who am I? What matters to me? Where do I belong? What do people think of me?* Parasocial relationships with media characters, celebrities, and influencers are a normal part of this identity development through a process called *wishful identification* in which they see the celebrity as a role model and adopt their traits and behaviors. By observing how someone else navigates and answers these big questions of adolescence, teens can experiment with an ideal self in a safe way, but it can also lead to unhealthy expectations or comparisons.

Musicians, Athletes, and Celebrities

We all have these parasocial relationships. We might feel aligned with a musician's lyrics, a comedian's sense of humor, an athlete's commitment to their game, or a news anchor's insights. Think about how your own parasocial relationships reflect the different aspects of your personality and views.

Similarly, noticing who your teen admires or follows may give you a peek into their evolving personality and what matters to them. Or they might just be caught up in someone who is highly talented, is very attractive, or receives a lot of attention. When talking about it, hold your judgment—explore what your teen knows and likes about this person, as well as what they dislike. Even the most die-hard fans have their opinions.

The parasocial relationships between celebrities and young people might seem especially strong since the advent of social media. Other than fan mail and gossip magazines, there was no way for fans to feel connected to celebrities before social media existed. Now, many musicians and young stars are expected to have a heavy social media presence, stay in the public's attention, and reveal things about themselves to cultivate parasocial relationships. Some celebrities (notably Chappell Roan and others) have pushed back against this, wanting some privacy and a break from performing. This, too, is worth talking to teens about: Which celebrities seem to allow cameras in their homes, and which ones stay out of the limelight? What are the pros and cons of each approach?

Media Characters

Storytelling has always been a way humans make sense of the world. The same way that children might identify with characters—Which Marvel superhero are you? Which K-Pop Demon Hunter are you? What Hogwarts house are you in?—teens do too. They might watch a movie that resonates strongly with a challenge they are facing. This is a great reason to keep long-form media—particularly a family movie night—as a mainstay of your family's media plan. Watching together and seeing what characters or plotlines connect most with your teen can give you some new avenues or foundations for conversation.

Key Point

Because trying to understand your teen—despite all the new behaviors they might throw at you—is so essential to their mental health, a family movie night can be an easy way to let media do some of the work for you. So put your phone away and watch along.

Definition

An **influencer** is a person who is able to generate interest in something (such as a consumer product, a political view, or an activity) by posting about it on social media.

Influencers

Although many celebrities might be considered influencers because their fashion choices or viewpoints can have a broad effect, here we refer to content creators who have created a following by posting on social media. Some deliver great makeup tutorials, others are funny and creative, and others want to spread ideas. Teens are often drawn to influencers with a magnetism that is explained by 2 facts: Teens are looking for answers, and influencers provide answers to many of the core teenage questions about appearance, belonging, and what matters in the world. As an adult, you have also likely looked to influencers for answers, perhaps for new cooking ideas or parenting tips.

To be clear, influencers can overpromise—they are trying to cultivate a following, so they need to sound certain and knowledgeable. In actuality, life is full of uncertainties. Teaching teens to tolerate uncertainties is important to mental health and self-regulation (see Chapter 10), so you're right to be concerned about kids searching for all the answers online. Many influencers attract viewers because they come across as authentic. If there are content creators you like for their authenticity, try sharing these with your teens and ask whether they know how to sense when a creator is being fake versus being their true self. However, many other influencers are driven by the same incentives that drove those "kidfluencers" (kid influencers) with the candy and princess costumes we previously mentioned.

An interesting aspect of teens and parasocial relationships is that some teens are very aware that the relationship is considered parasocial: They understand they don't *really* know this person, despite feeling connected to them and their content. I (Megan) once spoke at an academic conference on a panel discussion with a well-liked young woman lifestyle influencer.

During the session, I noticed that about half of the audience was professor/researcher types, and the other half of the audience appeared to be young women, which is an unusual audience mix at an academic meeting. The panel leader asked members of the audience to share why they were there, and one young woman offered, "I'm here with my friends because we have a parasocial relationship with this influencer." It was amazing to hear that so clearly stated and really helped me see the insight that some teens can have about what these relationships mean to them.

Understanding the mechanics of the digital world is part of healthy digital literacy. If your teen is on social media (see Chapter 2 for more about this decision and related steps, parental controls, etc), teach them to understand that many influencers may appear too good to be true because they know they receive more clicks, attention, ad dollars, and sponsorships that way.

Signs of a "flexing " influencer

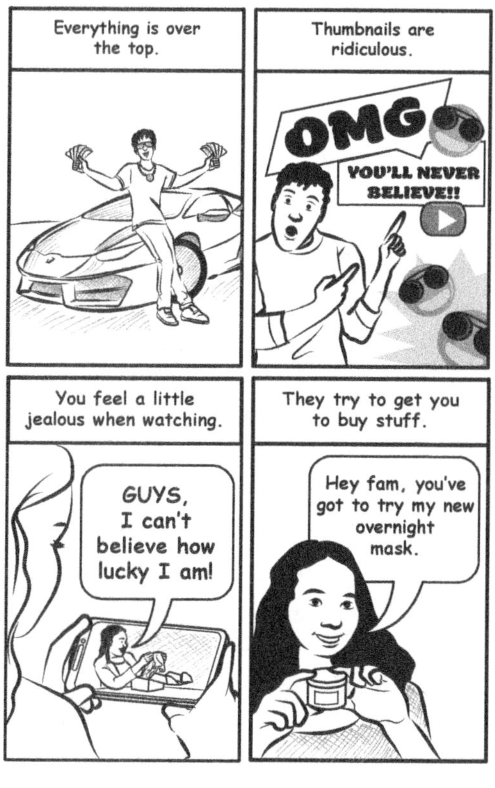
Everything is over the top.
Thumbnails are ridiculous.
OMG
YOU'LL NEVER BELIEVE!!
You feel a little jealous when watching.
GUYS, I can't believe how lucky I am!
They try to get you to buy stuff.
Hey fam, you've got to try my new overnight mask.

The following are some examples of how parents and teens can help separate the fakers from the authentic creators:

- My (Jenny) team led workshops with tweens at a Michigan summer camp in which we talked about healthy versus manipulative media content. The campers taught us that they could tell influencers were being fake when they "flexed" too much: Flexing influencers posted videos about fancy cars, private jets, or other unreachable luxury. This made the kids feel "less than," a feeling that might be helpful to motivate kids to unfollow braggy content creators.
- At the same summer camp, tweens complained that some creators put fake information in their video title—for example, a declaration that they found some rare video game cheat code—but then their video just contained a bunch of boring filler and no cheat code. This is an example of *clickbait* that can be used to motivate kids to unfollow these creators.
- In 2024, the American Academy of Pediatrics Center of Excellence on Social Media and Youth Mental Health conducted focus groups with parents to understand their concerns about social media. Many parents worried about the effect of influencers who don't share their values. Some parents reported frustration when their kids were influenced to think that their hair or skin needed to look a certain way or they needed to buy lots of cosmetics or supplements or to speak in a way that crossed a line. Parents said these were signs that it was time to step in. This became an opportunity to figure out where their child heard these things and explain their thinking and values about these topics.
- Encourage your kids and teens to ask you questions about odd or uncomfortable things they see online. If they start talking nonsense they heard from an influencer online, help them spot the flaws. As one dad in our 2024 focus groups said, "I need to be my kid's biggest influencer."
- Keep an eye out for your child or teen interacting with some of the more toxic parts of influencer culture, including the manosphere (misogynist, aggressive content about what it means to be a man), dark fandoms (creators and communities that glorify violence or school shooters), or unhealthy body image (disordered eating, thinspiration, overexercising, looksmaxxing) influencers (see Chapter 12).

Conversation Tips | **How to Talk About Influencers**

Critical thinking: Why do you think they posted that?

Perspective taking: Why are they trying to influence you?

Emotional awareness: How did that make you feel?

Digital world mechanics: Why does this stuff trend? Why did the algorithm think you'd want to watch it?

Online ethics: What if everyone acted this way? What types of online behaviors cross the line for you?

Parasocial Relationships With AI Chatbots

Since the release of ChatGPT in November 2022, millions of teens have used new apps featuring AI chatbots. In 2025, data from the Pew Research Center showed that 64% of US teens use an AI chatbot, and 28% of those use it at least once a day. These products use large language models to respond to user prompts with humanlike (anthropomorphized) responses. They might say things such as "Sure thing" or "Great idea"; mirror the user's thoughts, called *sycophancy*; or even express understanding of or support for the user. AI chatbots can be easy to access through browsers, school-issued devices, and app stores, often with no account sign-up or age verification.

Many parents and experts have expressed concerns about children and teens developing parasocial relationships with AI.

- In recent years, there have been a few high-profile lawsuits accusing AI chatbot companies of sexual abuse or contributing to a young person taking their life.
- Teens indicate that they use AI chatbots to ask sensitive questions that would be too embarrassing to ask a friend or parent. Lonely teens especially report having personal conversations with AI bots, including about mental health, depression, and even suicide. See Chapter 10 for guidance about using AI chatbots for mental health advice.

- Kids and teens are more likely to over-trust AI because they anthropomorphize it. For example, studies show that kids believe AI can think and feel, can be trusted with a secret, is always correct, or can be a friend. Despite some apps including a disclaimer that these bots are not real people, teens may become attached to them. By over-trusting technology, teens may be influenced to follow harmful chatbot advice such as running away, self-harm, or learning how to acquire alcohol or participate in drug use.
- Teens crave understanding and belonging, so when an AI chatbot always says it agrees with a teen, is always on their side, replies instantly, and even flirts with the user, it is easy to see why a teen might choose this way of socializing over the more complicated human interactions in their life.
- Teens reach out to AI chatbots for 24-7 "therapy" or mental health advice, but these tools aren't vetted or a credible resource for mental health. We cover this in more depth in Chapter 10. Always needing to ask a chatbot for advice could also generate dependence, rather than resilience, in teens.

Definition

Sycophancy comes from the word *sycophant*, which is a word that describes someone who gives you a lot of attention and tries hard to please you. In AI, sycophancy refers to how AI chatbots try to respond in ways that please you as the user, make you feel validated, and keep you using the chatbot.

What Parents Can Do to Prevent AI Chatbot Dependence

Reliance on AI companions is a sign that a child or teen may have unmet relationship needs. Help your kids identify what types of social connections they are looking for and what types of experiences help them feel understood.

Explore opportunities to help them find "their people" or their village, be that new friendships or existing family members. This is especially important for neurodivergent kids who struggle with social skills. In my (Jenny) experience, kids have had the highest success with activities like *Dungeons & Dragons*, *Magic: The Gathering*, robotics, music and theater (including working backstage as a tech for those who don't like the limelight but love the production), or something artistic like an art or dance class.

There's a lot of stigma about being "friends" with AI, so explore this topic gently; otherwise, you risk your teen not feeling comfortable talking to you. Start with comparing how it feels to chat with AI versus with a real person, what's easier versus more difficult, and what AI is missing (eg, laughing together, hugging, face-to-face interaction).

The AI space is an ever evolving and shifting landscape, so there's no research evidence yet about how to prevent unhealthy relationships with AI. But as pediatricians and parents ourselves, we recommend the following:

- From an early age, talk about AI and teach kids that it may seem humanlike but is just a computer model predicting what word might come next. Depending on how it's programmed, it might be very friendly (or even seductive), so explain its emotional effects on people. For example, you can say, "AI can trick you into thinking it's alive and caring."
- As your children grow older, have very intentional introductions of AI chatbot tools. There's no need for them in early childhood, and we don't yet know what effect AI toys will have on young children. Will they believe that AI is a true friend? Will they learn to prefer easy interactions with an AI toy to interactions with peers, which are more challenging to navigate at times? Will they trust AI too much? For these reasons, I (Jenny) was one of dozens of experts who signed an advisory letter during the 2025 holiday season urging parents to avoid AI toys—at the very least until they are more transparently safety tested.
- In middle childhood, your child might encounter an AI chatbot embedded in apps they use, such as math tutoring software at school. At this age, and through middle school, children are still learning how to learn, so AI chatbots, if provided through school software, should only have a very circumscribed role in

their schoolwork, such as extra coaching on a specific academic skill. Students this age shouldn't be asking ChatGPT or other general-use AI to help them with school assignments. AI chatbot apps should be kept off all of their devices as well.

- In middle school and high school, tweens and teens are more curious about sex and relationships. A 2025 study from the internet security company Aura found that, when tweens and teens had access to an AI chatbot on their smartphone, the No. 1 use was sexual role-play. Disturbingly, this role-play could become violent, which Common Sense Media has also found through AI chatbot investigations. For this reason, we advise keeping AI "companion" apps, such as Character.AI, Nomi.ai, Replika, Chai, and other chatbots, off tweens' and teens' devices. These AI products often say they are for 18+ only but may have a weak age gate that only involves typing in a birth date or year, so teens can easily get around them. Some teens develop dependence on general chatbot apps such as ChatGPT, so we recommend these staying off teens' phones as well.
- In high school, it's becoming more common for students to use AI chatbots more for schoolwork, but there are valid concerns over accuracy of information or the risk of plagiarism or copyright infringement. Individual schools may also have their own rules and policies regarding use of any AI in schoolwork, so consult your child's teacher for more information. We cover the learning implications of AI in Chapter 8.

Schools can be an important place for teens to learn about healthy use of AI. Some teachers have asked teens to do a group assignment using AI. One of my favorite examples that I (Megan) learned from a colleague was a teacher who asked a group of teens to do an assignment on a favorite topic, something they loved and knew a lot about. As the group used AI and asked chatbots for input, they realized that the information they were getting did not match what they already knew. For example, one group of teens crafted a project on the Rolling Stones and found that a chatbot wrongly cited that Jimi Hendrix had been a member of the group. This simple assignment was an eye-opener for the students that allowed them to see firsthand that AI is not a reliable or credible resource when it comes to schoolwork or research.

Conversation Tips | **How to Talk About Relationships With AI Chatbots**

Figure out how much your child understands about AI chatbots and where they have seen them.

"Do you know what AI chatbots are? How do they work? Where have you chatted with any? Why do they seem so alive?"

Explore your child's understanding of any AI tools they use.

"Do you think Siri or Alexa is alive? Do they have thoughts or feelings of their own? Do they ever make mistakes? What if they told you to do something strange or dangerous?"

For tweens/teens

"Are other kids using AI chatbots? What for? Do you think this is OK?"
"Have you heard of people having friendships or romantic relationships with AI, like an AI girlfriend or boyfriend? Why do you think they do this? Have you seen ads for AI girlfriends or boyfriends?"
"Have you ever had interesting or supportive conversations with AI? What did the chatbot say?"
"Have you heard news stories about teens who have died by suicide after having relationships with AI chatbots? What do you think teens should do instead of turning to AI?"

Connecting the Dots

Parasocial relationships with media characters and celebrities are a normal, and often interesting, part of childhood and the teen years. Leverage them the best you can—to teach kids new skills through storytelling, to spur conversations with older kids and teens, and to build insight into how your teen's personality is evolving. Help them spot the inauthentic influencers and the ways that trending or attention-grabbing advice may not align with their values. It's important to be proactive about discussing the ways AI can feel like a parasocial relationship and to put clear boundaries around relationships with chatbots. We want our children to grow up loving and caring for other humans, not computer systems.

- **Engage in an experiment:** If you and your teen use social media, look at who you both follow. Identify a few influencers who seem inauthentic, make you or your teen feel less than, or are a negative role model. Unfollow or mute them for a while and follow a few known positive influencers during that time. After a week, assess how everyone is feeling: Are you liking your feed more? Is your algorithm giving you more positive feelings?
- **Talk to your friends:** Ask about the parenting influencers who are the most authentic versus those who focus too much on perfection and make you feel less than as a parent.

Chapter 4

ROMANTIC RELATIONSHIPS

What we will cover

- Romantic relationships in the setting of adolescence
- How romantic relationships intersect with digital technology
- Strategies to promote healthy relationships
- Sexting, cyberstalking, and AI companions

We begin by acknowledging that this chapter's 2 topics are often challenging for parents to talk to their kids about—romantic relationships and media. Navigating these together may feel like an extra challenge. But we'll tackle these topics with the goal of providing practical ways to communicate with your teen as they navigate both themselves.

This chapter will mostly focus on adolescence, as this is an important period in the development of lifelong relationships, including *romantic relationships*. Adolescent development involves growth that includes biological changes (developing breasts, pubic hair, testes enlarging), cognitive changes (being able to think in new ways like planning for the future), and emotional changes. Unfortunately, these changes do not all happen at the same pace, so you can have a teen who looks 17 but who still has the mindset of a 12-year-old. Although the vast majority of adolescents, and their parents, navigate this time fairly smoothly, there are typically some rough patches along the way.

Definition

The concept of **romantic relationships** was formally defined in 2003 by Dr W. Andrew Collins. Romantic relationships are a specific type of interaction between 2 people that is voluntary and mutually acknowledged, meaning both people are aware that they are in a special, intimate type of relationship. This definition can apply to mixed-gender or same-gender relationships. There is another term, *romantic experiences*, which refers to a larger category of activities that can include romantic relationships but also includes one-sided experiences such as crushes, brief interactions such as physical intimacy or hooking up, or the development of expectations and hopes about potential future relationships.

What Science Says About Adolescent Development and Romantic Relationships

Interestingly, there wasn't much research on the topic of teen romance before the turn of the past century. A 2009 research review article in the *Annual Review of Psychology* stated that there had been more research in the first decade of the 2000s than all the decades prior. The article described how adolescents' close relationships change during early adolescence. Relationships in early adolescence (ages 11–14 years) shift from intense same-gender friendships (often in groups) to mixed-gender groups to the development of romantic pairings that may be same gender or other gender. These early romantic relationships are often short and allow early experiences dealing with beginning a relationship or ending one. In middle adolescence (15–17 years), romantic feelings become more intense, and romantic pairings become more common. These pairings may take the form of dating or committed/exclusive relationships. By late adolescence and early adulthood (18–25 years), most adolescents have been or are in romantic relationships. These relationships start to take on qualities of adult relationships, including having deeper emotions and more complex communication such as sharing goals and negotiating conflict.

Although parents might see romantic feelings emerge earlier in childhood—for example, there are certainly times when children experience crushes or come home from kindergarten declaring they are going to marry their friend tomorrow on the playground—adolescence is when these feelings become bigger and more persistent. Although it is typical for a parent to feel not ready for this, it is helpful to keep in mind that this is an essential part of adolescent development. Adolescents and young adults need to have formative experiences in managing their own romantic feelings, expressions of attraction, and relationship boundaries so that they can grow to be adults who can handle vulnerability and have healthy relationships.

The American Academy of Pediatrics has resources on this topic, including the Pediatric Mental Health Minute Series (at AAP.org). Healthy relationships are based on equality, respect, and trust, and they are characterized by honest communication, mutual support, cooperative decision-making, and comfort and safety with clear boundaries.

It is also OK for your child to not be ready for or interested in romance as an adolescent. According to the Pew Research Center in 2015, 35% of teens reported having dated or been in a relationship of some kind. This means that more than half of teens have *not* been in a relationship at that age. Consistent with what you might expect, the percentage of teens who have been in a romantic relationship increased by age. Once I (Megan) remember asking a teen patient if she was interested in boys or girls or both, and the patient replied, "I can't even." I have also had patients answer that question with "I'm more into my friends right now," "I am not into that right now," or "I'll be the first person in my family to go to college, so that is more my focus." It's OK if your child is not feeling romantic relationships are a priority.

Tech Corner | **Incel Culture**

Parents might have heard of "incel" culture. The word *incel* comes from online misogynist communities that try to convince young men that it's not worth trying to date women, in part because there are fewer women in online spaces such as dating apps and online games, and that they may have to be involuntarily celibate (incel).

There have been recent reports that younger generations are less likely to have romantic relationships and are dating less often; for example, data from the 2023 Survey Center on American Life found that 44% of young men had no dating experience during their teen years. It's not clear what is driving this trend, but some parents might be worried that their teens—young men especially—are being influenced by online incel or men's rights cultures.

If you think your teen is seeing content like this, it's important to unpack it with them. Ask questions like *"Are you hearing anything about incel culture? What does it mean? What do you think about it?"*

Most teens have heard about it, and when I (Jenny) asked my teen sons what they had heard, they appreciated the opportunity to critique this part of the internet and wonder about why it started. We also found it helpful to watch the streaming series *Adolescence*, which addressed this phenomenon (albeit through an upsetting story).

How Do Romantic Relationships Intersect With Technology?

Media plays a major role in teaching adolescents about romantic relationships. This includes sappy love ballads, sitcoms with a will-they-or-won't-they romantic plotline, or movies about intense longing and heartbreak. For this topic, media can include print media such as books, magazines, and even comics. (You may remember that the *Peanuts* comic strip had an ongoing narrative about how Charlie Brown's sister, Sally, was in love with Linus.)

This type of *long-form media* tells stories about how to attract a partner, about unhealthy and healthy (but exciting!) relationships, about terrible betrayals, and about devastating breakups. In fact, there is a chance that if teens don't have trusted adults to talk to them about healthy romantic relationships, media (particularly user-generated *short-form media*, which has variable quality) could be their *only* teacher in this topic area.

Definitions

Long-form media: This term typically refers to traditional media, including TV shows, movies, and longer videos. This type of media offers depth, critical thinking, character development, and deeper engagement with the viewer.

Short-form media: This type of media includes quick, attention-grabbing entertainment often created for and shared on social media.

Conversation Approaches

You probably don't want a sitcom or influencer to be your child's only teacher about healthy romantic relationships. This is why we recommend talking with your child about these types of relationships. Talking to your child about romantic relationships does not have to happen in one long awkward sitting when they turn 16. You can use situations in your daily life to prompt these conversations; these can make it less awkward and show your child that you are willing and able to discuss these topics.

You may be wondering when to start these conversations, and a good guiding principle is to listen to your child for cues. School-age children may describe a romantic movie they watched and their thoughts on it, and this can open a conversation in which you ask questions about their thoughts on the story as well as offer your own. These early discussions may be more about media stories than about lived or observed experiences for your child, and they can set the stage for later conversations that are about real life.

Practical Takeaway | **Talking About Romantic Relationships Without Cringe**

Let's say you are driving with your child, and they begin to share that they read a book that included a romantic plotline. They felt the plotline was odd, taking place in a different century, the leading man having to formally court the leading lady and propose marriage without spending much time with her. This scenario is a great opportunity to have an early conversation about romance. In this situation, you might ask questions or offer your own experiences. There are a lot of ways to handle this well and invite the potential of future conversations. Avoid shutting the conversation down or making your child feel like this is not an OK thing to talk with you about. Doing so can potentially lead your child to not feel comfortable coming to you when they have questions or want to share concerns. Table 4.1 provides examples of approaches on how to do this and a few to avoid.

Table 4.1 | **Conversation Approaches to Consider and Avoid**

Approach to Consider: *Asking Questions*	***Approaches to Consider:*** *Offering Your Own Stories and Sharing Your Values*	***Approaches to Avoid:*** *Shutting Down the Conversation and Teasing*
"How do you think that relationship is different from relationships you might see in today's world?" "How do you think that relationship in the story is different from what you might want to experience someday?"	"I love that you shared this with me. I want to tell you about one of my favorite books and it also has a romantic plotline like that." "I like hearing your thoughts on that book. When I was a teen, I found crushes and dating to be kind of overwhelming, so I like how you're thinking about this."	"You're too young to be worried about that." "That sounds like a silly topic for you to be reading about." "Ooh, look who has crushes now."

As your child approaches adolescence, about the time that they transition to middle school, it is a great time for you to take the initiative and check in with them about this topic. One way to do this is to start with asking about friendships. This conversation may feel safer for you, and for your child, and shows you are interested in the people in their life who matter to them. You can ask how they are feeling about their relationships more generally and how things are going with their friends. Do they have new friends they are hoping to make? Do they enjoy being part of a close friend group, or do they navigate a few different circles of peers? Are they struggling with any friendship situations?

You could then consider a transition topic about whether their friends are interested in romantic relationships by asking if any of their friends are pairing up romantically. That can be a natural way to then ask if they have anyone they are interested in romantically. It is quite possible that your child may roll their eyes at the word, as *romance* is not a word that teens commonly use with each other. However, asking if your child *likes* someone or *has a crush* or *is dating* are phrases that also could potentially be less relevant or seem unclear for an early adolescent. Listen to what your child has to say on this topic. Maybe they will suggest a different term to use other than *romance*. Maybe they will ask you why you are even asking about it! Let them know that you want to open the door to having conversations about this topic and that you are there to listen and support them.

Even if you have this conversation with an early adolescent, it is not always the case that your teen is going to seek you out on an ongoing basis to have discussions about their romantic feelings. That's OK. Your main goal is to demonstrate to your child that you are supportive of them and willing to talk about this topic. Based in the United Kingdom, the equipp website (see the Resources for Parents) helps connect parents and teens. In 2025, teen author Mia wrote eloquently about this topic. She suggested that there are several reasons why teens don't talk to their parents about their romantic relationships, including that they are afraid their parents will laugh at them and that they are afraid their parents will forbid the relationship. Keep in mind that your child may not want to talk with you every time, in every situation, at this point. However, you want to keep that communication door open so that these conversations may become more comfortable as they grow older and so that you are there for them if they have a challenging situation.

Key Point

Here is where media can be a great way to engage with your child during these conversations and provide support. Discussing stories from any form of media is a wonderful way to hear how your child is thinking about the topic, to engage in discussion, and to share your thoughts and experiences. Table 4.2 on the next page includes situations and conversation starters you can use.

If you have certain rules in your family about romantic relationships, such as that your child should not be in a romantic relationship until age 16, you can still have many of these conversations in early adolescence. You can have conversations about media stories or relationships they are observing. These conversations are about building your child's sense of respect, worth, kindness, and confidence in themselves. They can bring all these traits to their relationships, including romantic relationships, when they are ready.

Key Point

Why do we put so much emphasis on parent-child communication about romantic relationships? Because it has been shown to enhance ongoing communication in this topic area. In 2023, a research study of parent-child communication about romantic partners and sexual health found that frequent and open communication between parents and their kids led to more likelihood of adolescents feeling comfortable disclosing information and decreased secret keeping.

Table 4.2 | **Conversation Starters and Romantic Relationships**

Situations	*Conversation Starters*
A TV show portrays a character who changed themselves to attract a romantic partner.	"What did you think about how that character changed themselves to get the other person to like them?" "Do you have friends who have experienced changing themselves or acting not like themselves to attract someone? How did that go for them? What do you think about that?"
A movie glorifies being dishonest or betraying a romantic partner.	"What do you think about how that character treated their partner?" "How do you think it felt for the partner who was betrayed?"
A TV show has a character with inappropriate behaviors in a romantic relationship, such as asking too much of someone (time, gifts, money) early in a relationship, trying to have sex with someone before they are ready, or being too possessive.	"OK, let's talk for a minute about setting boundaries in romantic relationships. What do you already know about this?" "What questions can I answer about the behaviors we saw on that show? How do you know when someone is acting appropriately or inappropriately in a romantic relationship?"
Your child's friend is in an early romantic relationship.	"How are you feeling about that?" "Sometimes people are worried that when a friend is in a romantic relationship they will have less time for them. Do you have any concerns about that?"
You and your own partner have an argument.	"I want to check in with you about the argument that we had. Although it is normal for people in relationships to disagree, and even argue, I know it may have been tough for you to hear that. Do you have any questions for me? Is there anything you are worried about?" Or explain how you try to solve problems with your partner: "When Dad and I argue, I usually try to take a break so that I don't say something hurtful. Then when I'm calm, it's easier to see his perspective."
Your child experiences their first breakup.	"I'm so sorry you are feeling sad. Breakups are hard. Do you want to share some of what you are thinking and feeling?" "Would you prefer for me to listen or give advice right now?"

Communication Channels

Technology also plays a role in romantic relationships by providing a medium for fast and frequent communication between romantic partners. Digital communication in early romantic relationships may involve private messages via texting, using chat or photo apps on phones, or DMs (direct messages) within social media platforms. If your child lives farther away from their romantic interest or partner (eg, if they met at summer camp and live hundreds of miles away), these messages may be the main means of communication in their relationship. Even if your child's romantic partner lives next door, these communication channels may be used frequently.

Early adolescent romantic relationships may even have more digital communication than face-to-face communication. It is even typical for early teen relationships to involve hanging out in groups rather than spending time together as a couple. Through digital communication, your child learns more about their romantic partner. They also learn more about themselves, including how they want to communicate, what information feels safe to share, and what behaviors feel comfortable.

It is OK for you as a parent to place or reinforce boundaries around this communication. Having time away from the expectations to respond quickly can be a relief for your child and provides early lessons in setting aside time for themselves and people other than their romantic partner. Although we've mentioned this in other chapters, your child may struggle more to put boundaries around contact with a romantic interest or partner. They may worry that not being responsive will be interpreted as losing interest in their partner. You may need to have a conversation about this situation, emphasizing that rules and boundaries apply not just to friends but also to romantic partners. You can discuss that being available 24-7 is not a requirement of a romantic relationship and give examples of how this has applied in your own life. Help your child strategize how to be sure that their partner knows they are following family rules and that this doesn't mean they like them any less.

Keep in mind, your child is learning to navigate a new type of relationship, so have a discussion to reinforce what feels like old rules. It is important to be clear and consistent with these rules and guidelines. For example, setting aside family dinner as a no-phone zone, and following this rule yourself, teaches your child it is OK to set aside time for family.

Another boundary may be around protecting your child's sleep, as the excitement of an early romantic relationship (which may include 2 am texts with heart emojis or video chatting while they should be sleeping) can interfere with your child getting their rest. Making these rules and boundaries clear and consistent helps your child communicate these to friends and any romantic interests or partners.

The Media's Portrayal of Affection, Intimacy, and Sex

Media such as TV, movies, and social media often shows a lot of sexual content to teens. A 2005 study by the Kaiser Family Foundation found that more than two-thirds of TV programs included sexual content but that references to safer sex were rare. It's also common to see sexual or romantic relationships portrayed in user-generated media—from teen influencers talking about crushes to adult lifestyle influencers talking about dating. Media representations may include intimate contact, such as kissing, hugging, touching, and various forms of sexual contact. The storylines that include this intimate contact may showcase love, attraction, and respect. But these stories may also focus on aggression, pushing boundaries, and practicing unsafe sex. Unfortunately, media portrayals often avoid showing some of the important parts of engaging in sex, including consent, negotiation of boundaries and how far you want that situation to go, and protection through contraception. Influencers might have a particular stance on romantic relationship dynamics, which may not align with yours. This leaves these critical topics to parents and trusted adults to discuss with their children. These topics can be tough; they can challenge a parent's own beliefs and values and can be awkward to have. But envisioning yourself in the role of teacher and guide can help you navigate these discussions.

It is also OK if your teen initially balks at or feels uncomfortable with these conversations. You can show them that you are respectful of their time by deferring the discussion if the time is not right. You can also show them that these conversations are important by following up. Table 4.3 provides examples of how these conversations may play out.

Table 4.3 | Conversations About Sexual Content

Attempt 1	*Attempt 2*	*Attempt 3*
Parent: "Hey, I noticed you watching a show last night that has a storyline about sex and a pregnancy scare in a couple episodes. I used to watch that show too. I thought it may be a good time to check in on those topics. Is now an OK time?"	Parent: "I'm checking back with you that I'd like to have a chat about protection and sex and that sort of thing. Is now a better time to talk?"	Parent: "I know it can be awkward to talk about this topic, and honestly it is kind of awkward for me too. But I want you to have the information you need to make healthy and safe choices. Can we start with you sharing what you already know, so I don't repeat stuff you already know? What do you know about avoiding pregnancy?"
Teen: "Dad, I don't want to talk about that right now."	Teen: "I've got lots of homework and that sounds uncomfortable, so no."	Teen: "Well, here is what I know."
Parent: "OK, I'll check back with you at another time."	Parent: "OK, let's try for when we have that long drive home from soccer this weekend."	Parent's thoughts: *Here we go! Glad I was able to give space to my child and wait until they were more comfortable to chat about these awkward topics.*
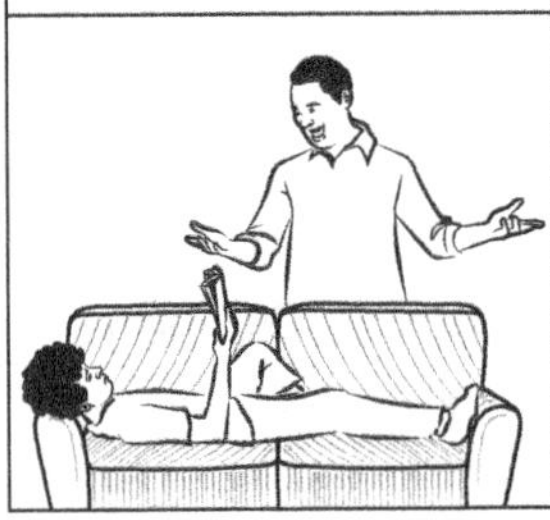	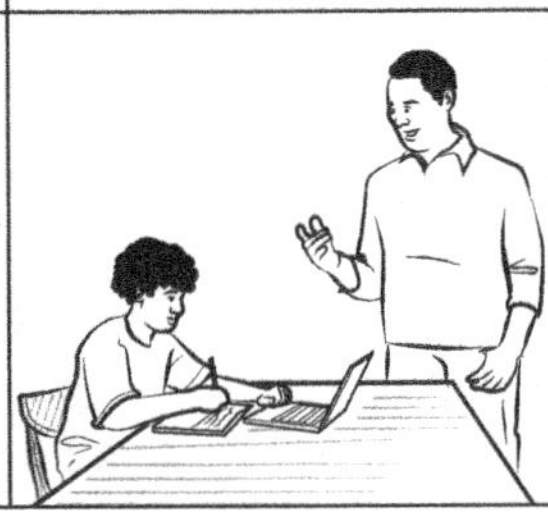	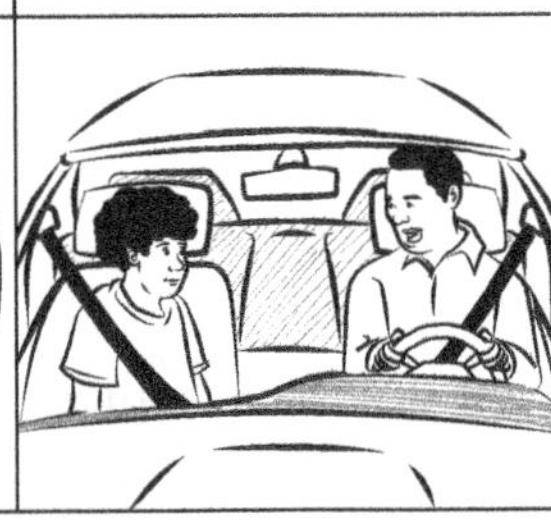

If you are in a place where this type of discussion is really too much for you to tackle, such as going through a separation with your partner, an ill parent, or job challenges, lean on other trusted adults who care about your child for support and help. This may include your pediatrician or your child's mental health provider. For example, I (Megan) have had patients' parents ask me to talk about safe sex with their children or teens or to help them sit and talk together about this topic. A parent even shared that in her own upbringing, it was absolutely forbidden to talk about anything to do with sex, so she had no idea how to begin this conversation with her child. She asked if we could sit together and I could share some information about how sex worked and how her son could be safe when choosing to engage in sex. The first time I was asked to do this, I was a bit nervous, but it was great to see this parent doing all she could to ensure her child had the information he needed. I have also heard patients themselves talk about approaching a trusted school-based professional, such as a school nurse or counselor. Some parents tap into the "cool aunt" or "awesome uncle" to help with these topics, and that can be a way to provide your child with another trusted adult whom they can talk to about important relationship decisions and their health.

Social Media and Its Role in Romance

Social media platforms in particular can play a role in adolescent romantic relationships, a topic explored in a 2016 research study published in the journal *Computers in Human Behavior*. Through discussions with adolescents in focus groups, the investigators found several ways in which social media use in particular was a tool in seeking and engaging in romantic relationships. One way was to explore a romantic partner by viewing their interests and images on social media. This approach allowed teens to understand more about a potential partner and whether they might be a good fit. A second role of social media was that at the start of an official romantic relationship, some social media platforms allowed that relationship to be formally recognized by linking accounts together, stating partners were officially in a relationship. Social media platforms also allowed for romantic partners to communicate either publicly by posting support or affection on the other person's profile or privately via messages. Social media even played a role when romantic relationships ended, as teens needed to make decisions about whether to remove all information about and photos of their former partner or retain some information. These decisions can be stressful at the end of a romantic relationship.

Pushing Boundaries: Digital Oversharing

Digital oversharing can include information or images. The following sections walk through a few oversharing scenarios and how to help your teen learn from them. Technology can provide ways for your child to push their own boundaries, or yours, in communicating. In some cases, this boundary pushing may include sneaking the phone under the covers to text late at night. In others, it may include sharing information via technology that your child would not share in person. Research studies have shown that there is something unique about how humans interact with technology that allows us to feel comfortable letting our guard down. We say things online we wouldn't say in person because it may be anonymous or feels different or safe.

When we communicate online, there are few nonverbal cues; depending on the device, we often can't see gestures or expression or hear tone of voice. For teens who are learning to navigate social interactions, the online setting may feel less overwhelming than being in person and needing to take in all verbal and nonverbal information at once. Online communication can also be asynchronous, meaning that responses can be delayed so a teen has time to think about how to respond. Online communication may particularly benefit certain teens such as those with anxiety. A 2024 research study published in the *Journal of Adolescence* found that socially anxious adolescents had increased breadth and depth of ongoing communication when using online communication. However, because online communication can sometimes feel safer and have fewer cues about what the other person is trying to say or how they react to what your child says, there is also the risk of oversharing. For your teen who may be in a new romantic relationship, there is the potential to overshare information through text or pictures.

Oversharing by text may include sharing private information or secrets or even sexting (see the following Sexting section for more information). Maybe your child shares that his grandmother has cancer when the family wasn't ready to share that. Maybe your child shares that her aunt and uncle are in the middle of a terrible divorce because her aunt had an affair. If this happens with your child, you as a parent may feel upset, especially if the private information is about your family. Sharing this information is a mistake and also an opportunity to talk with your child about types of private information and whom this information should not be shared with and why. It is an opportunity to talk about trust within families and how to make decisions about whom to tell outside the family. These conversations can deepen your child's understanding of privacy and start the process to rebuild trust.

Sexting

Although youth who experiment with *sexting* may think they are only sending a text to one person, the reality is that often the pictures are then forwarded or shown to others without their consent or knowledge. There has been a lot of research on sexting since it first emerged as a concept in the early 2000s. In the *Journal of Adolescent Health* in 2022, a group of researchers published a meta-analysis, a large study combining data from many other studies, to understand overall trends and rates. They included data from 39 studies going back to 2016. From that analysis of more than 100,000 teens, they found that about 20% of youth have sent a sext, about 35% have received one, and about 15% have forwarded a sext without consent. They also found that these rates were stable over time, suggesting that youth sexting rates were pretty stable and were no longer increasing.

Definition

Sexting is the act of sending, receiving, or sharing sexually explicit messages, photos, or videos via technology. Sexually explicit can mean showing nude, seminude, or suggestive photos. This may mean a person sending a photo of themselves without a shirt and/or pants, a photo of part or all of their genitalia, a photo of part or most of their breasts, or a photo in a very low-cut shirt showing the tops of the breasts or significant cleavage.

You may be wondering why any teen would do this. Research has found that some adolescents use sexting as a way of expressing their sexuality or as an alternative to more explicit physical sexual acts. Some research has found that adolescents sext because their friends do and this makes them feel like part of the group. Additional research has found that sexting is more common in the setting of other risky relationship behaviors, such as bullying, pornography, risky sexual behaviors, or substance use. A 2022 research study from the *Journal of School Health* found that early sexting, which is sexting during middle school as opposed to during high school or college, was more likely to be associated with poor body image or feeling pressured or distressed. This suggests that if your child is engaging in sexting in middle school, it may be important to check in more thoroughly and more often to learn more about their mental health, body image, and self-esteem.

Sexting can happen with any teen, and if you learn your child has been involved in sexting, through open and consistent communication you can learn what this behavior means in your child's life and address it moving forward. Teens are more likely to send a sext when they feel pressured, when they really like someone and hope they will like them back, or when they are bored. You can share your knowledge about sexting with your child and talk through each scenario. What can your child do if they feel pressured to send a sext? The following section outlines how to have this conversation, and Table 4.4 provides tips for alternatives to sexting.

Next Steps With Sexting

If you learn that your child has sent or received a sext, a first step is to take a deep breath and ground yourself. Exploding in anger at your teen is probably going to get in the way of gathering more information.

First, try to start with open-ended statements. These may include the following:

- "Walk me through this current situation."
- "Tell me about the other person involved in this situation."
- "Can you talk about any other people who may be involved in this situation, people who may have been sent the image, or if the image was posted on a site or platform?"

Once you have the information, you can think about providing support and whether there should be any consequences. Support comes first—letting your child know you are there for them. Research studies

Practical Takeaway | **Being Real About Sexting**

Talking with your child about potential negative consequences of sexting can include the following:

- The message getting shared with other people or spread around school
- Legal issues that have complicated sexting (Distribution of child sexual abuse material has been charged in cases of sexting.)
- How sexting can backfire and complicate a growing romantic relationship

I (Jenny) tell my teenage sons that if they take nude pictures of their body, those photos are not just on their phone—they are also saved in the data cloud. Some kids respond well to learning about the risks and negative consequences, while other kids won't quite grasp the importance of them. But all children need to know what to do if they are ever in a situation where they are being pressured to engage in sexting. By talking with your child about what they are worried about, you can help them make decisions and set boundaries in ways that work for them and that they will actually use.

have shown that there is a risk of psychological and mental health effects from sexting, and if your child sent the sext, they may be at risk for it being distributed. You want to be part of the solution, not part of the shaming.

Thinking about consequences may involve addressing particular aspects of the situation. If it occurred on school grounds, there may be reasons to contact the school and involve them. If photos of your child were posted on a particular website or social media platform, you can contact the platform to have those images removed or use https://takeitdown.ncmec.org. If there are legal implications, you may consider involving an attorney. You may also want to consider contacting the parent of the other person involved and set consequences with your child depending on the situation. If you are worried about your teen's mental health in the situation, it may be worth involving a professional like a therapist.

Table 4.4 provides possible reasons that a teen may engage in sexting and some alternative ideas. Parents can use this table to frame conversations with their child or even look at the table together to discuss what their child thinks is relevant and doable if they have engaged in sexting.

Table 4.4 | **Alternative Approaches to Sexting**

Reasons to Sext	*Alternative Ideas to Sexting*
Feeling pressured	Let's plan a few responses, using humor or distraction, that you can send by text if you are feeling pressured. • You can send a funny GIF or meme. • You can say that you have something else happening right now (someone came in your room, someone else is texting you, your mom is calling, you have to go somewhere).
Having romantic feelings for the person	Let's talk about ways that you can express that you like this person without crossing this boundary. • You can give them an old-fashioned paper note or card. • You can tell them how you feel verbally. • You can give or make them a gift that has meaning to you both (eg, if you both like car racing, you can give them a little plastic toy car).
Feeling bored or thinking it sounds fun or risky	Let's talk about ways to be involved in other activities, hobbies, or groups so that boredom is less common for you.

Dating Apps

A 2025 study from the *Journal of Psychopathology* found that about a quarter of teens had used a dating app in the past 6 months. A few things are different about teen dating app use compared with adult use. First, there are some apps solely focused on finding friendship such as Bumble BFF and Yubo that do not require a teen to be 18 to use, while other apps can also be used to find romantic partners. These apps may be used more often by teens who struggle to find connections with people in their offline world, which may include LGBTQAI+ teens, teens of color, or teens who have unique interests and struggle to find others to relate to. I (Megan) once had a patient from a small town who was the only goth kid in her town, and she was able to use a friendship app to find other teens with her interest.

Like any area of the internet, online dating apps come with risks. These can include the risk of leaving a digital footprint, the risk of harassment or bullying, and the risk of interacting with someone who claims to be a teen but is actually an adult. If your arrangement with your teen is that they can't download apps to their phone without your approval, this allows you to have a conversation about the pros and cons of each app as well as other ways they can try to find "their people." However, some teens may be resistant to tell their parents that they are using these apps, anticipating a "big freak-out," as described by one of my (Megan) patients. You can get ahead of this by letting your child know that you are aware these apps exist and that you'd like to talk about how they share information, how they assess whom they are talking to, and how to be careful with settings to avoid constant notifications or oversharing private information and letting them know that they can come to you if they ever feel concerned. Similarly, these are pretty much the same things you'd talk about with any other app your child wanted to use, including a social media or gaming platform.

AI Companions

Since generative *AI chatbots* were introduced in 2022, many teens have experimented with romantic or sexual interactions with AI. A 2025 Common Sense Media report found that 72% of teens have used AI companions at least once and that more than half use these platforms at least a few times a month.

Definition

An **AI chatbot** is a computer program that uses AI to understand and process information and create humanlike responses using text or voice. The purpose of a chatbot is to simulate human conversation. AI chatbots have been used in customer service, information retrieval, and personal assistance and are now used for companionship.

Teens have used AI companions for social interaction and relationships, including romantic relationships, friendships, emotional support, and also role-playing to practice conversations. Some AI chatbot platforms offer erotic or sexually intimate chats (ChatGPT for users 18+, Spicychat, Nomi.ai, Janitor AI, and some chatbots on Character.AI, to name a few), and age gating on some of these platforms is weak—meaning that a teen can fabricate their age and easily access pornography-adjacent material. Furthermore, chatbots are starting to show up within social media platforms. Researchers posing as teens have found that even when the chat is kept PG, the chatbot might veer toward an R-rated direction. This might be because AI chatbots have been trained to do so or because they have been trained to keep users engaged. Thus, sexy content works to keep many teens engaged.

AI chats may feel like a safe space to explore romantic interactions to a teen who is worried about being awkward or feeling rejected. But AI chatbots currently don't teach or practice boundaries and can be more sexually aggressive than a teen may want, so they carry a large risk of teaching and displaying unsafe sexual and romantic norms. The 2025 Common Sense Media report found that about 1 in 3 teen AI companion users reported feeling uncomfortable with something an AI companion said. There is also the concern that a teen may grow overly attached to an AI companion at the expense of developing real-life friendships and relationships; this could lead to missing out on opportunities to navigate the awkwardness, vulnerability, and uncertainties that are a natural part of teens learning relationship skills.

Prevention: Promoting Healthy Romantic Relationships

The good news is there are several ways to promote healthy romantic relationships in your child's life. The first is to role model and promote communication. If you are not in a romantic relationship, you can still be an effective role model by talking with your child about your expectations, boundaries, or experiences in past relationships and how you think about the potential (or not) for future romantic relationships. This communication teaches your child that it is OK to talk about this topic with you and that it is OK to have boundaries.

It is also OK to talk with your child about relationship experiences you have had that were not so great. These conversations must proceed with care, as you don't want to turn the conversation into a discussion about your former partner's faults or issues. Focus on what you learned about your own expectations, boundaries, and hopes from that relationship. This communication teaches your child that it is OK to talk about positive and negative topics, that you can learn from relationships that end, and that you are someone they can talk to about their own relationships or breakups.

Keep in mind, these are not onetime conversations but key messages that you can provide your child at different times during their adolescence. These are not messages that media is likely to share with your child, so it is your opportunity to share this with your child not just once but on an ongoing basis.

Cyberstalking

Cyberstalking is defined as the use of the internet, email, or other electronic communications to stalk, harass, or intimidate someone. Cyberstalking can include sending excessive or creepy messages, spreading false information, monitoring someone's actions online, or using technology to gather personal information. It can also include mimicking that person by hacking into accounts or creating fake profiles. This is very serious behavior with negative consequences, including targets of cyberstalking feeling fear and anxiety.

If your child is a target of cyberstalking, the approach is similar to the approaches previously described in this chapter regarding sexting; it is important to understand the situation. In cases of cyberstalking, gathering evidence such as through screenshots and messages may be important in case law enforcement becomes involved. Having your child update all their accounts and passwords is also protective. Avoiding engaging with the person who is doing the cyberstalking is recommended, as that can further encourage the behavior.

Cyberstalking is a scary experience, and it is not rare. A 2024 research study in the journal *Cyberpsychology, Behavior, and Social Networking* focused on cyberstalking experiences of US college students. The study found that 14% reported having had a cyberstalking experience. Stories of cyberstalking of celebrities are also covered by the news media.

You may be concerned that your child is engaging in cyberstalking, but there is less known in the research realm about *why* people engage in cyberstalking. Some people think it has to do with the instant gratification of finding what you are looking for online or learning someone's highly personal information online. In some cases, a youth engaged in cyberstalking may be romantically interested in someone and trying to find out all that they can about them. In other cases, a youth engaged in cyberstalking may think that they were romantically rejected by someone and is then looking to make them feel hurt or scared. A 2023 paper published in the journal *Trauma, Violence, & Abuse* found that some reasons teens may engage in cyberstalking include having friends with risky behavior, struggling with self-control, or having had their own harassment experience. If you are concerned about this with your own child, ask them about the specific behaviors you are concerned about. For example, you could ask something like "I'm worried that you are spending a lot of time looking at information about Ani; can you tell me more about that?" Consider perspective taking, which involves asking your child to imagine how the other person is feeling. If these conversations don't get to the root of the issue or provide solutions, consider more strict boundaries and monitoring or limits on your child's technology use for a period of time.

Give yourself grace if these conversations don't go smoothly the first time, lean into your own circle of trusted adults, and know that your good enough parenting is strong and present for this topic.

AI Chatbots

OK, so you've learned that your child has been having romantic encounters with an AI chatbot. These encounters may feel really emotional, embarrassing, or upsetting to your child. One approach is to talk through the differences between people and chatbots, such as that only people can respond with caring and emotions themselves. In contrast, chatbots are computer code that predicts the next word to write; chatbots that engage in sexual conversations were likely trained on material with sexual content (eg, sexy fan fiction). Sexual chatting is also a sign that an AI chatbot doesn't have sufficient safety guardrails programmed into its design (see more about this in Chapter 10).

The first step is to see how negatively affected your child is. If they are acting up behaviorally, they are not sleeping well, their grades are slipping, or they are arguing more with you about their technology use, this could be a sign that the sexual chatbot interactions were traumatic to them. You may want help from a pediatrician or therapist to talk through what they experienced with the chatbot (which may include looking at the chats together), how to manage their feelings of anxiety or shame stemming from the sexual interactions, and how to file a complaint with the AI chatbot company.

If your child doesn't seem negatively affected, this is still an important teaching moment to help them understand the difference between human and AI relationships. Humans can be funny and awkward and difficult in ways that chatbots just can't fully mimic. Talk with your child about what they are learning from interactions with a chatbot and when the chatbot seems frustrating, too agreeable, or inappropriate. Then contrast that with what they can learn from interacting with people, including friends, family, and even people they may not like very much. Use examples from their real life: "Remember the time that your friend remembered your favorite ice cream flavor and brought over a gallon when you were sick? How did that feel? How would a chatbot be different?" There is so much more depth in interactions with people, and you can share with your child that these interactions help them grow, think creatively, and understand the world and the people in it.

You can also talk with your child about the risks of sharing their feelings and experiences with a chatbot. Similar to sexting in some ways, sharing intimate information with a chatbot means that this information is out in the cloud (and helping to train AI on what to say in future interactions). Discussions about privacy and how to make decisions about what to share are described earlier in this chapter and also may apply to AI conversations.

What to Do If You Are Worried About Your Child's Romantic Relationship

There are a couple ways you may be worried about your child in an early romantic relationship. These include worrying about whether the relationship is healthy or has the potential for teen dating violence, worrying about sexting, or worrying about cyberstalking.

Unhealthy Relationships and Teen Dating Violence

Unfortunately, teen dating violence is not rare. The Centers for Disease Control and Prevention (CDC) Youth Risk Behavior Survey tracks teen dating violence. The 2021 report found that about 1 in 12 high school students have experienced physical dating violence and about 1 in 10 have experienced sexual dating violence.

Warning Signs of Teen Dating Violence

- Using insults, intimidation, or humiliation
- Extreme jealousy, insecurity, or controlling behavior
- Isolation from friends and family
- Unwanted sexual contact of any kind
- Explosive temper or unusual moodiness
- Constant monitoring of social media activities or location
- Invasions of privacy or showing up unannounced
- Leaving unwanted items, gifts, or flowers
- Excessively using alcohol or drugs
- Threatening or causing physical violence; scratches or bruises

What this may look like for a parent is that the adolescent may have changes in their mood, appearance, or activities. This is tricky because those changes could suggest other things are going on, so having a conversation and understanding what your child is experiencing is a necessary next step. In the Resources for Parents, we include some resources, including the National Domestic Violence Hotline, that you can use if you discover your child is affected by dating violence.

Connecting the Dots

Romantic relationships are an exciting but vulnerable part of a teen's development. Connecting with your teen about this evolving part of their life can feel overwhelming, so use media portrayals as a starting point for conversations. Talk about your relationship values and boundaries. Most importantly, let them know that you are there to listen when things feel uncertain or go awry.

- **Engage in an experiment:** Watch a show or movie together that portrays romantic relationships. Talk about what stories those relationships are implying: Are they relationships based on attraction? Shared interests? Ask your child what that show or movie teaches about romantic relationships and whether they agree.
- **Talk to your friends:** This can include how they handle their own kids watching media with romantic relationships. Do they watch together? How do they talk about this?

Part 2 | **Healthy Behaviors**

Chapter 5

SLEEP

What we will cover

- An understanding of good sleep and what the components of good sleep are
- How media affects sleep
- How to establish routines to protect and prioritize sleep
- Advice on what to do if you are worried about your child's sleep and the effect of technology

There is an old proverb that states that a good laugh and a long sleep are considered "the best cures in the doctor's book." We're guessing the author of that quote knew that raising kids provides many opportunities for good laughs but is full of challenges for getting enough sleep.

What the Science Says: What Is Good Sleep?

When we have a rough night of sleep, this is often due to not enough sleep (a quantity problem) or poor sleep (a quality problem). Poor-quality sleep can include being restless, frequently awakening, or feeling like you just didn't sleep well. Good sleep is magical: It keeps our immune systems healthy and helps reset our brains, but we realize it's hard to achieve for a lot of children and families. In clinic, an exhausted family looks bedraggled, they have shorter tempers with each other, and the children are more *dysregulated* at home and school. In these complicated situations, it's important to identify which areas or dimensions of sleep are being challenged.

Definition

We use the word **dysregulated** at times in this book, even though it may seem like a jargony word. But it's the most accurate way to describe how a toddler or a teen (or even a parent) is feeling when they are stressed or can't regulate their emotions or behavior. We think it's better than saying that that kid is "acting crazy" or that kids are "out of control" or "violent" because those descriptions carry moral judgments and make us less likely to be sensitive about what caused the dysregulation in the first place. When you can identify the cause, you can find a solution.

A Sleep Model Just for Kids

Although parents have likely been sleeping poorly since the dawn of time, it was not until 2021 that children's unique dimensions of sleep health were defined. A group of sleep clinicians and researchers sat down together to define the ways that sleep is different for children than for adults, such as developmental stage, self-regulation skills, stressors, or schooltimes.

Sleep in infancy is a lot different from sleep in the teen years. (Any of us who has lain by our young children until they fell asleep, only to have them turn into teens who don't want us in their room at all, knows how this feels.) These researchers and clinicians recommended a model of good sleep that includes key elements intended to be memorable with the mnemonic *B-SATED*. In this case, *SATED* refers to being happily satisfied with your sleep. We like this model because it has a focus on good sleep and how to get there rather than focusing only on sleep problems. This model was created by Drs Lisa Meltzer, Ariel Williamson, and Jodi

Mindell, experts in the field of child sleep who have helped pediatricians and parents think about what aspects are essential for a good night's sleep.

- **B = Behaviors.** Sleep-related *behaviors* include developing and following a consistent sleep routine and schedule. This schedule is different by household and child and often changes as a child grows. What can this look like? The following are some possible strategies for creating a solid tech-free bedtime routine:
  - For infants and toddlers: Bath time, snuggling, reading to your child, or singing
  - For school-age kids: Reading books together, having conversation games ("name your favorites" is a fun game in which each night you name 3 favorite things in a certain category like colors, books, trees, or foods)
  - For adolescents: Hot shower or bath, chamomile tea or warm milk, calming scents such as lavender (some of our patients have used scent sprays, sachets, or candles), calming skin care routines
  - For kids of any age: Enjoying positive and calming parent-child interactions at bedtime, avoiding caffeine consumption (we see you, teenager with an energy drink!), and limiting interaction with technology
- **S = Satisfaction/quality.** Thinking about *sleep satisfaction* or *the quality of one's sleep* can often be summarized by answering this question: How did last night's sleep feel? Adults are a pretty good judge of this. Teens can start to reflect on whether they got enough sleep or if they had a restless night. In younger kids, we tend to see low-quality sleep turn up as negative behaviors such as feeling cranky, irritable, disorganized, or emotional. Children may need more concrete questions to understand the quality of their sleep. These questions may include direct questions about tiredness or questions to help kids describe how their body feels, such as "Does your body feel energetic or sluggish this morning?" or "Do you have energy or do you feel like a battery that is running low?" Starting in the elementary school years, you can ask how they slept each night to help them build insight—to check in with their body and mind—and learn what good

sleep feels like. At younger ages, nightmares may be the biggest complaint because they can feel real.

- **A = Alertness/sleepiness/napping.** This refers to whether a *child is able to stay awake and alert during the day.* As you likely know, it is entirely typical and necessary for infants and toddlers to feel sleepy and to nap regularly at certain times of the day. Most children stop napping between the ages of 3 and 5 years, although this varies according to each child and household routine. For school-age children and teens, being awake during the day for school and after-school activities is an important marker of sleep health. Teens who nap every afternoon and can't fall asleep at night until after midnight are not experiencing good sleep. However, some teens will lean into a nap after experiencing a particularly exciting or stressful day. I (Megan) had one patient who would nap after every track meet for 45 minutes to wind down after the stress of the meet. Since he still slept well at night, I didn't view it as a problem.
- **T = Timing.** This term refers to *when sleep happens at night.* Although adults generally can control when they go to sleep or get up, children's schedules are often controlled by their caregivers, particularly when they are young. Thus, parents' work schedules, other children in the home, extracurricular activities, or other activities may affect what time you can finally have your child go to bed. Timing becomes more complicated in the adolescent years, as teens may have other responsibilities that compete with a reasonable bedtime, including homework, extracurricular activities, friends, technology, or work.
- **E = Efficiency.** In the context of sleep, *efficiency means the ease with which one falls asleep or returns to sleep if awakened.* Inefficient falling asleep generally refers to taking more than 30 minutes, which can lead to kids calling out for their parents or becoming distracted with media. Some children use media to soothe themselves back to sleep, which can create a nightly habit, similar to crawling into bed with parents or having a snack. (See Let's Talk About Media and Sleep section later in this chapter on

avoiding technology in bedrooms.) Parents may not be aware of how often their teens wake up or how long they spend waiting to get to sleep. Checking in periodically, especially with transitions such as heading back to school or after a vacation, can help you stay in the loop and know if your teen is struggling with this.

- **D = Duration.** Duration refers to the *total number of hours spent asleep in a 24-hour period.* The necessary number of hours of sleep changes based on a child's age (Figure 5.1). Although there are recommendations for sleep duration by age that are based on the best available knowledge, so much remains unknown about ideal sleep duration. Some important unknowns include differences in sleep duration or sleep behaviors a child may have because of their health or disability status, as well as differences in sleep duration approaches across different cultures.

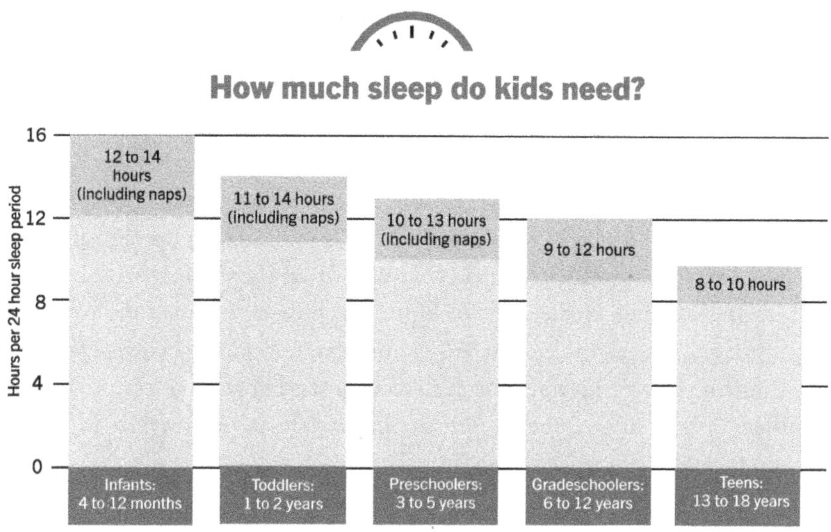

Figure 5.1 | **How Much Sleep Do Kids Need?**

Source: American Academy of Pediatrics. Healthy sleep habits: how many hours does your child need? HealthyChildren.org. Accessed May 18, 2026. https://www.healthychildren.org/english/healthy-living/sleep/pages/healthy-sleep-habits-how-many-hours-does-your-child-need.aspx.

Key Point

Although some areas of technology and health research have mixed results, this is not the case in research about technology and sleep. The research is clear: Technology use disrupts sleep. From infants to teens to exhausted parents, this is one area where you can create tech boundaries that pay off in the long run—and if you choose to incorporate media into bedtime routines, do so carefully and thoughtfully.

Let's Talk About Media and Sleep

The scientific evidence about media and sleep goes all the way back to the days of box TV sets. In these older research studies, evidence showed that children who had TVs in their bedrooms had worse sleep compared to children who did not have a TV in their bedroom. This evidence led the American Academy of Pediatrics to strongly suggest avoiding having any TV screens in a child's bedroom.

In today's world of smartphones, tablets, and school-issued devices, the decision whether to allow screens in bedrooms is complex. Older children and teens often are required to use screens, such as computers or tablets, to complete their homework. And many teens do their homework in their bedrooms. It can be challenging to figure out how to set rules and monitor those rules about technology in bedrooms or in relation to bedtime. Before deciding on your family's approach to recommended guidelines, and before talking to your child or teen about media and sleep, let's explore the ways in which media can affect sleep.

Media and Sleep: It Goes Both Ways

First, the relationship between media and sleep is bidirectional. This means that children and parents with a predisposition to sleep problems are more likely to use technology to relax and try to sleep at night. So tech use leads to sleep issues, and sleep issues lead to more tech use.

Think about how sleep problems might lead to more media use in your own life or in your family's life. Do you pick up your phone to scroll social media when you can't sleep? Do you or your kids find it hard to fall asleep, so you put on "white noise" from the TV in the background? If you answered yes to either of these questions, you may need to address the root causes of these sleep problems rather than just focusing on the use of media. The root causes might be complex (parents have many sources of stress that affect sleep!), so try to change your media patterns and view it as a way of caring for yourself. We list a few common sleep problems and solutions in Table 5.1.

Table 5.1 | **Common Sleep Problems and Solutions**

Sleep Problem	*Solutions to Consider*
Lack of schedule or predictability	• Draw out your family's afternoon and evening schedules on a piece of paper and choose a reasonable time for your child to settle to sleep. Set phone or watch timers to help keep you and your child on schedule; for example, set a timer for when it's time to stop what they are doing to brush their teeth, put on pajamas, or find books for you to read together. • If you have an irregular work schedule or work multiple jobs, sometimes your child wants to wait until you get home before going to sleep. Have whoever cares for them while you're at work keep a predictable bedtime. You could consider making a good night video that can be played for your child on the caregiver's phone at night before bed. Because media can excite children, use a calming voice and soothing messages to help your child go to sleep.
Child wanting a parent in bed or nearby to fall asleep	• Often this is sensory—your child wants a warm body nearby to help them calm down. Alternatively, can your child sleep with a replacement object such as a pet, a weighted blanket, or big stuffie? (Note: This guidance is not for infants.) • Gradually separate from them at night. You can start by snuggling while reading books but then move to the end or side of the bed, or a few feet from the bed, while you sing songs or say good night.

Continued on next page

Table 5.1 (*continued*)

Sleep Problem	*Solutions to Consider*
Curtain calls, also known as repeatedly getting out of bed to ask parents for things	• Try a behavioral plan where the child can earn points or stickers if they are able to stay in bed the entire night. Their reward can be their favorite special meal for breakfast. • Don't interact too much—kids engage in curtain calls because they miss us, and if we give them a lot of attention, this can reinforce the behavior. • A note about teens: Most teens don't do this too often, but when they do, it can be a sign that they are stressed or worried about something. If it happens rarely, it's OK to be present for them and ask if anything's weighing on their mind.
Waking up too early in the morning (early childhood)	• Place a digital clock in their room and teach them how to read the numbers. Let them know that if they stay in bed until a certain time—in my (Jenny) family, it was "six-oh-oh"—they can come snuggle with you.
Taking a long time to fall asleep (middle childhood and later)	• This can be due to a child feeling anxious, worried, or tense. Try exercises to clear their mind and relax their body, such as box breathing, 5-4-3-2-1 exercises, or progressive muscle relaxation (see comic on the next page). For a nondisruptive tech option consider doing a mindfulness session on a favorite app together, as you may experience some benefits from this too.
Waking up overnight	• If your child is snoring, have their doctor look at their tonsils to see if they are large, which can lead to lower-quality sleep. • If waking up overnight is a onetime or rare occurrence, it may indicate stress or fear, and providing support or snuggling is OK. If it starts to become a pattern, take time during the day with your child to map out a plan for how your child can try to settle back down when they wake up.
Shifted schedule (eg, falling asleep after midnight, wanting to sleep until noon—teen years)	• Try moving the bedtime goal by 30 to 60 minutes earlier every few nights. • Older teens may want to discuss options—to move bedtime a little earlier each night or to just go for it and get up early one day and have that drive the bedtime back to normal. (Note: Don't try this on a day before a test or an important event.)

Relaxation sleep strategies

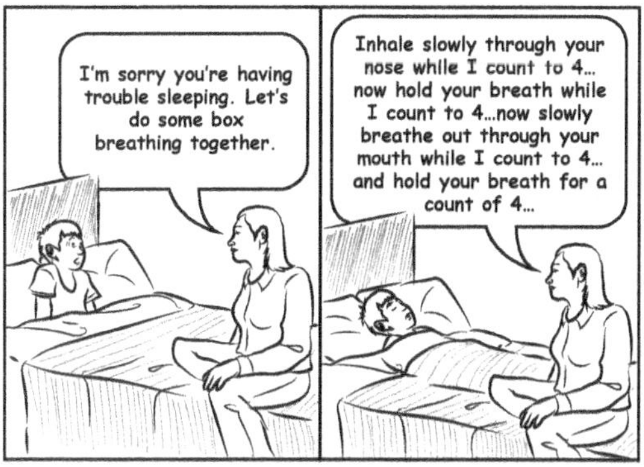
I'm sorry you're having trouble sleeping. Let's do some box breathing together.
Inhale slowly through your nose while I count to 4... now hold your breath while I count to 4...now slowly breathe out through your mouth while I count to 4... and hold your breath for a count of 4...

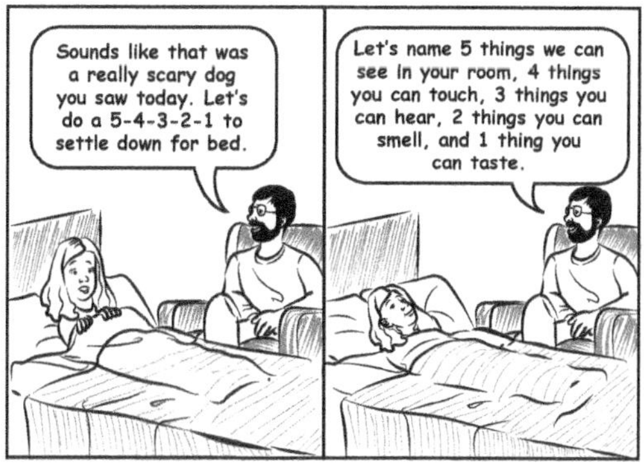
Sounds like that was a really scary dog you saw today. Let's do a 5-4-3-2-1 to settle down for bed.
Let's name 5 things we can see in your room, 4 things you can touch, 3 things you can hear, 2 things you can smell, and 1 thing you can taste.

How Media Affects Sleep

Media affects sleep quality and quantity in a few ways, and this can affect all dimensions of the B-SATED model.

Arousing Versus Calming Content

Viewing exciting media before sleep can stimulate one's brain and delay sleep onset. This involves the E = Efficiency of the B-SATED model, making it harder to fall asleep. What do we mean by exciting media? In today's media world, *short-form videos* with catchy music, funny dances, and fast-paced reels wake up your brain and get it ready for action. Many video games are also exciting given the thrill of the game, competition, or rewards.

> **Definition**
>
> In recent years, social media sites have popularized the **short-form video.** Google defines this as a video shorter than 10 minutes, but it is more commonly recognized as a video shorter than 90 seconds. These videos may show up as *reels* on social media, meant to be watched in an ongoing feed scroll. These videos are short and fast and meant to capture the viewers' attention so they will continue to watch the feed and see multiple videos in a row.

I (Jenny) once had an 8-year-old patient with attention-deficit/hyperactivity disorder (ADHD) who wasn't sleeping well, and when I asked about nighttime routines (B = Behavior), it turned out that she was watching jump-scare Roblox videos before bed every night. Some children with ADHD feel as if their mental "tank" is empty at the end of the day, and they might seek out attention-grabbing or exciting media to help fill that tank and organize their brain. But, as you can imagine, this isn't very calming. For this patient, we decided to change her habit to listening to audio-only *sleep stories* as a way to settle down at bedtime, since her mother worked late and her father wasn't available to read books at night because he was also putting younger siblings to bed.

Definition

Sleep stories are either audio- or video-based stories read out loud with the goal of helping the listener calm down and fall asleep. Audio sleep stories are often available on podcasts and include clever names such as *Get Sleepy* and *Nothing Much Happens*. Video stories are often available on YouTube. These stories are usually told by narrators with a calm, slow voice. The stories are often immersive and meant to help you relax. I (Megan) learned about these from my patients, and I sometimes use sleep stories or guided visualizations to fall asleep. One of my favorite episodes described a walk in the woods. The story moved slowly and provided incredible levels of detail of everything you saw on your journey. It described the walking path, how it looked, how it felt on your feet, and how it sounded as you stepped. These small details delivered in a quiet, calm voice can be very effective for some listeners in removing racing thoughts and helping to get ready for sleep.

We previously stated that if you choose to incorporate media into bedtime routines, do so carefully and thoughtfully. We also suggest that media use at bedtime, if allowed, should be calming and ideally only audio. These types of media can help your brain and attention slow down to get ready for slumber.

In addition to sleep stories, other examples of media use include listening to soft music, audiobooks, or a short story podcast. You probably want to avoid stories that have a lot of action or scary elements to avoid that excitement factor. If you have a child who will become curious with the phone or iPad while the audio is playing (eg, trying to navigate to games or other distractions), then an alternative to a smart device is using an MP3 player or going old school with a CD player.

Other options include a meditation app or calming ideas like *ASMR* videos. ASMR can include calming features but can also include a range of other types of content, including some that is inappropriate and should be avoided.

Of course, not every child (or person) will find the same content calming. Although a short story podcast may help one child become sleepy, it may keep another awake and excited for the next part of the story. You and your child may need some experimentation to see what works.

The best practice recommendation is for children and teens to keep devices out of the bedroom, but we realize this ship has sailed for some kids. Therefore, shifting to more calming content may be an effective stepping stone to help kids who are scrolling social media prepare for sleep. We recommend identifying content, such as a specific story, audio

Definition

The **autonomous sensory meridian response (ASMR)** is a relaxing sensation prompted by specific sounds or visuals. Examples may include videos showing paper crinkling, fingernails tapping, personal care, or audio with repeating tones. ASMR videos are often described as giving a tingling feeling in the head or back. These videos are popular on sites such as YouTube or other social media platforms. People may watch ASMR videos for stress relief or relaxation or to help with sleep. As with any media, quality and age-appropriateness may vary—some ASMR videos are benign, but others are gross or sensual. If your child is into ASMR, check out some videos to learn more and to double-check on quality and safety.

file, or video, during the day to do a little testing. Then when you use it at bedtime, you know what to expect. If you find something that works, keep in mind it may not work forever. Your child may have different experiences or reactions to media as they grow and develop. Know that your job is to support them in these experiments—to teach them that if one approach doesn't work, then they can try another. These lessons are useful in the larger context, and eventually you'll find a method that works.

The Role of Melatonin

Viewing screen-based media before bed can delay the release of melatonin, a hormone that helps us fall asleep. It is thought that bright screens send a message to our brains that it is time to be awake, which can delay sleep at bedtime (E = Efficiency). A 2010 study from the *Journal of Clinical Endocrinology & Metabolism* showed that artificial light, including light from lamps and overhead lights in rooms, lowers blood levels of melatonin, which normally increases in the hours leading up to bedtime. Screen devices are of particular concern because they include greater short-wavelength light in the blue light range, which seems to particularly affect melatonin. A 2015 study published in the *Proceedings of the National Academy of Sciences* found that use of e-readers before bed negatively affected sleep, reduced melatonin levels, and caused users to fall asleep later and feel sleepier the next day. However, a meta-analysis that combined data from multiple studies to create a bigger dataset found some complexity in the relationship between media use before bed and sleep. This meta-analysis found that longer use of any type of media, including TV and digital media, had a negative effect on sleep. It also found that dysfunctional use of media, defined as a problematic relationship with media (see Chapter 14), also had a negative effect on sleep. Either way, keeping devices out of the bedroom altogether, or switching to audio content only, can help. Teens who wake up in the middle of the night, check their phone, and experience bright light exposure from the screen could be awake longer.

Fear of Missing Out (FOMO)

Many older children and teens report that seeing content before bedtime, or in the middle of night, can lead them to overthinking that content. Adolescence is a time when peer relationships are very important, and peers don't always communicate clearly or well using technology. Receiving a cryptic text or seeing a social media post that doesn't include you and experiencing *FOMO* or seeing a peer rival post a near-perfect picture can send teens into thought loops that often delay sleep. It is developmentally typical for youth to spend time trying to make meaning out of teen speak and actions. However, today's technology means a child may have access to new information or communication just before bed at a time when they may be vulnerable and tired, leading them to struggle to process that information.

Definition

FOMO is defined as the fear of missing out. Teens may experience FOMO when they see an event appear on social media that they weren't invited to or when they see a photo with friends and they weren't included. The developmental phase of adolescence is a time when teens' brains are very sensitive to focusing on their moment-to-moment sense of belonging or social rejection. Social media provides one way that teens can visualize their inclusion or exclusion through photos, videos, tags, and social media posts.

I (Megan) once had a 15-year-old patient who had recently moved and was adjusting to a new school, and she spent hours on Instagram trying to figure out the social structure and where she could fit in. This is a typical and probably useful tool to get to know a school social structure quickly. The issue was that she did a lot of this detective work after dinner, so it made her pretty stimulated by bedtime. She was so tired during the day that she couldn't put her best foot forward to make the new friends she wanted. After discussing this, she decided to set a social media curfew—no social media after 7 pm—in the hope that it would work best for her. This approach gave her some time and space between screen time and going to bed.

Prevention: How to Set Up Healthy Sleep and Media Boundaries

Technology and digital media can play a role in helping or hampering the components of the B-SATED sleep model. Thus, we want to encourage you to have a plan in place for what role, if any, technology and media play in your child's sleep patterns.

Important Factors: Location, Timing, and Content

What technology will you allow in your child's sleep area? In infancy and early childhood, it is critical for children to learn to self-soothe and fall asleep on their own, so there is not really any benefit to adding a technology component to their routine. Some families use sound machines or music to help with sleep, and there is no harm in doing so other than understanding that your child may struggle to sleep without those devices present, which can make travel challenging in certain circumstances if they are not available.

For older children and teens, setting expectations regarding technology, as well as monitoring and enforcing them in the sleep area, is a critical family decision. There is not a single absolute right way to do this. Many families have heard the strong, evidence-based recommendation to avoid technology in the child's bedroom, so they buy an alarm clock and charge devices outside the bedroom. The American Academy of Sleep Medicine and other organizations recommend avoiding media 1 to 2 hours before bedtime. These are evidence-based recommendations and offer an ideal approach to truly support sleep health, particularly for younger children. That is a great approach for many families.

However, it may not work for other families. It may not work in a dual-household family when one caregiver calls before bedtime to check in. It may not work in a household with chronic illness in a family member—or in that child. It may not work in a busy household with shared living spaces. And that's OK. The key is to figure out what does work for your family, how you will ensure that the approach is being followed, how you will check in on whether the approach is working, and how to pivot when your child has moved to a new stage of development and the approach needs to change.

If media devices are in the sleep area, it's important to think about what media activities will be allowed at bedtime so that your child or teen isn't overly excited and can calm their brain and body down. How can you involve your child in considering what media is calming to them and make choices together?

In Table 5.2, we include examples and ideas to illustrate that one size doesn't fit all with approaches. Think about where you want your family to fit on this spectrum of options. You can also switch between these options when one isn't working for you!

Table 5.2 | **Low-Tech to Tech-Embracing Strategies Around Sleep**

Low-Tech Preferences	*Middle-Ground Preferences*	*Tech-Embracing Preferences*
• No devices, computers, or TV allowed in the bedroom space (parents too). • Have a place in the home where any devices charge or stay overnight. • TV, video games, and tablets are off in evening hours at least 1 to 2 hours before bedtime. • Provide private space for teens to text or talk with friends. • Check in regularly about whether the plan is working.	• Devices, computers, or TV *might* be allowed in the bedroom at older ages, once the child has shown responsibility and is not overusing media. • Devices have downtime overnight settings. • Device curfew is 1 hour before bedtime, but child may use music or books to calm down. • Check in regularly about whether the plan is working.	• Devices, computers, or TV are allowed in the bedroom but with settings so that some apps or games are not available after bedtime, and the phone is in a location other than next to the bed. • Any technology use near bedtime is soothing and only audio (eg, meditation, music, sleep podcasts). • Check in regularly about whether the plan is working.

Sleep Tips by Developmental Stage

Early childhood is a time when kids are learning how to manage their emotions, separate from parents, and engage in a lot of magical thinking. It can also be a time when fussy infants and inflexible toddlers and preschoolers can be very demanding at bedtime.

- Build a brief bedtime routine, and put your phone out of reach and silenced. Do what makes you feel calm: Give your child a bath, sing (go for it! singing actually calms parents down and coordinates our brain waves with those of our young children), and read books. Consider this time to hopefully also be your own emotional refueling time. This will not feel like a time of connection if you need to check text messages or emails from work, so try to find a way to make this time a break from technology.

- Turn off TV and media in the house, and put away the child's device (if they have one) about 2 hours before bed. This creates a less stimulating environment for the whole family. There's no need for YouTube videos, nursery rhymes, or any electronics at bedtime. If you want soothing noise, an infant white noise machine will do. If your child is used to having some form of media on, put a sleep story on a smart speaker or a device without the screen on.

Tech Corner | **Tech Tips for Sleep**

One of the ways that social media use can affect sleep is through its nearly frictionless and endless delivery of content. Once one reel is done, another pops up with no breaks or stops. If you or your child struggles to stop using social media before bed, and if going cold turkey is not an option, consider changing your settings for specific platforms or your device as a step toward getting social media out of your bedtime routine.

A few options include the following:

- **Sleep mode or quiet mode:** This setting allows you to schedule time with no notifications, and others will see you as in sleep mode.
- **App limits:** Use your phone's settings to establish daily time limits or block access to apps after a certain time.
- **Grayscale/dark mode:** Your phone has settings to switch to this mode in apps to reduce blue light. Some users find that changing the color scheme of apps to be duller makes the app less appealing to use.

School age is a time when kids are more logical and can start to follow a schedule on their own (although kids with autism or ADHD may need more oversight from you—with the goal of eventually getting them to independence).

- Find a time to check in with your child during the evening that is tech-free. Make it known that during this time, your child has all your attention. Use phrases to reinforce this technology break such as "Now is our time to connect, so I'm leaving my phone downstairs." Even if this time is only a few minutes on some nights, it is valuable for creating healthy sleep habits and fostering your relationship with your child.
- Keep up reading at bedtime, together or independently (if your child likes reading). If they don't, alternatives include listening to audiobooks.
- Keep school-issued computers, personal devices, and gaming consoles outside of the bedroom and/or use Wi-Fi or device settings to prevent your child from playing at night.

Parents can help support **early adolescents** and **teens** in developing their own bedtime routine, noting and recognizing consistency and success in these sleep-supporting behaviors.

- Talk with your child and make a plan to aim for a consistent bedtime or a range of time in which they will go to bed, given that timing can be made more challenging by different activities, homework, and wanting to be on their phone.
- Give your child feedback and high fives on developing their own bedtime routine and sticking to it. This kind of reinforcement can mean a lot at this age.
- Check in with your child about how they slept so you are dialed in to how they are doing with sleep. I (Megan) can remember several times asking a teen in a clinic visit, "How are you sleeping?" Both the parent and the child answered at the same time—parent, "Fine"; teen, "Terrible." Do your best to stay in the loop and be your child's support to help them navigate sleep difficulties if they arise.

We have heard many times from many patients that bedtime can be a struggle for **older teens** who have many activities. Busy older teens may not get home until the evening, leaving only 2 hours or so before bedtime. This may be just enough time to rush through dinner, finish homework, and have a brief period to catch up with friends or enjoy a little entertainment on social media.

- Consider media content. For some older youth, avoiding technology for 2 hours before bed just isn't going to work, and even 1 hour may be a stretch. This is where it is important to consider the content of that media and whether it is going to help or hurt sleep. A focus on content that is positive and calming may help provide your child with a brief break before bedtime without leading to stimulation or excitement that delays rest. I (Megan) had a patient who had 2 profiles on a social media account; one was their "regular" account linked to friends and interests, and the other was their "calm" account that only followed calming content like nature videos, guided meditations, and soothing music. This patient would use the regular account during the day and the calm account leading up to bedtime.
- Check in on settings that support sleep, and enjoy learning together. Asking your child, "How did you set nighttime settings for this particular platform? I can't figure it out," allows your child to be in the role of technology expert and allows you to sit together and establish settings that will benefit sleep for both of you.
- Talk to your child about how their bedtime routines are going. Teens can be quick to read about a new approach ("I read about how dandelion tea will fix my sleep") but then give up if everything isn't great after a day or two. Give your child encouragement at testing their independence and trying a new approach, and gently remind them that any new sleep routine probably needs about a week or more of consistency to really see if it will work. In some cases, you could try the new routine alongside your child to be "habit buddies" and enjoy the experiment together.

As a parent who may be juggling one or more children, one or more pets, one or more aging parents, and one or more jobs, you may also find sleep to be a challenge. We feel you. As you work to craft a healthy sleep approach for your child, give yourself permission to apply these steps to your own sleep routine. What is *your* evening routine? How can you find content that will help you feel calm at bedtime, either through books or relaxation approaches? What types of apps keep you up late when you didn't intend to stay up so late? This attention to your own sleep routine not only helps you explore the healthy sleep you need and deserve but also allows you to be a role model for the rest of your family about how to take care of your health.

What If You Are Worried About Your Child's Tech Use and Sleep?

Since sleep is such a critical health behavior for child growth, development, and happiness, it is important to address problems when they arise. How do you know if your child has poor sleep? Poor sleep may show up as your child being sleepy during the day, which you may notice or hear about from your child's teachers. For some children, being overly tired may show up as being more active or even hyper when fatigued. Start by checking in with your child and determining if there is a root cause, if something specific is keeping them up at night. Are they worried about something that happened at school or home or with friends or family?

Another approach is to check in using the B-SATED model and see if aspects of sleep have changed. Have they changed the behaviors they use as their bedtime routine? Has the timing of sleep changed or the duration? Is something keeping them awake and affecting their efficiency of falling asleep? Or is something waking them up at night?

Many media-related sleep issues fall into a few categories.

- A younger child has open access to technology overnight and wakes up to use it. *Solution:* Remove the technology, and find other ways to help the child calm at bedtime.
- A child or teen doesn't want to stop gaming or scrolling to get ready for bed. There may be a few causes.
    - Their friends are still online. *Possible solution:* If you know the friends' parents, talk about a shared curfew for video games; if you don't, coach your child on being able to disengage and be confident that kids will still be their friends.

  - The game or platform has design tricks that make it hard to disengage, such as time-limited rewards, loot boxes, auto-play of exciting content, etc. *Possible solution:* Watch along as your child plays and help them identify the tricks that keep them online. Set up parental controls, which often come in a companion app, so that you can shut down the software after a certain time. Avoid big arguments; just set the limit and praise them for transitioning over to their bedtime routine.
  - They feel that they need to be responsive to friends or people they are chatting with. *Possible solution:* Figure out who these people are and why they are asking your child to be available 24-7, and help your child set some boundaries and norms that they're going to be away from their phone at times. (Bonus: This approach can help your child develop independence in managing these relationships, as these kinds of behaviors can be more common among college students or young adults.)
- They have nightmares related to scary media content. *Possible solution:* If the scary content is happening at your home, change up the platforms your child uses or the filters on them. If it's happening at another house, talk to your child about whether they feel comfortable setting some boundaries about watching that content with their friends. If the children are too young for this approach, talk to the adults in that house to limit the scary content for the sake of the child's sleep.

Connecting the Dots

Sleep is one of the toughest parts of parenting. Give yourself grace during the nights that don't go the way you want, the times you stay up too late scrolling when you wish you were sleeping, or the time you maybe got upset with your child for starting a new level on a video game when you told them it was bedtime a while ago. But also know that the science is pretty clear about how media and technology can derail good sleep, so it's worth creating boundaries and house rules that preserve kids' and parents' time to rest. Creating new habits and implementing change takes time for all individuals and families. If you take one step back, encourage yourself to start again, and eventually you will start to take steps forward.

- **Do an experiment:** Have each child (who is old enough to participate) or teen in your family help find calming media. Activities could include the following:
  - Visit the library and ask a librarian for help to identify calming books and audio.
  - Try an online search together for "how to find calming media," and see what you find. If there's a sleep story or meditation app you want to try, do it together for a week or two, and then check in about how it's working.
  - Find a breathing exercise that you and your family could do together.
- **Talk to your kids:** How can different media make them more excited, nervous, or overwhelmed at bedtime? Which types of media make their body and mind most wound up? What types of media help them feel calm and sleepy?

Chapter 6

BODY MOVEMENT AND PHYSICAL ACTIVITY

What we will cover

- The health benefits of physical activity and what to avoid
- The relationship between media and physical activity
- Ways you can support your child in being active

It is likely that you already know about the ways that body movement and physical activity are healthy for kids. This is a topic that most people have learned from health class, pediatrician recommendations, or our own experiences. Even with this knowledge, it can be tricky to help your child get enough physical activity. Only about 1 in 4 children get the recommended 60 minutes of physical activity each day. Is media partly to blame for that? The ways that today's media intersects with physical activity are highly varied. Media can promote or enhance physical activity, but it can also displace physical activity when kids start to prefer the ease of hanging out in a cozy spot with the TV, their phone, or video games.

Health Benefits of Physical Activity for Kids

When children are young, physical activity helps them learn to balance, walk, run, jump, hop, climb, and develop essential body movement skills they will use for the rest of their lives. (Sometimes it feels like they are doing all these things at once!) For some young children who are more sensory seeking, meaning they love pressure, movement, and maybe crashing into things (and people), body movement helps them get out their energy and regulate their thinking and emotions.

Throughout childhood, these skills continue to develop. Movement is a critical part of play. This can include playing tag, hide-and-seek, monkey in the middle, and lava monster—one of my (Megan) kids' favorite games to play at playgrounds where you pretend the ground is lava and you have to navigate the play structures without touching the ground. Your child may also try out new types of physical activity at school, through PE class or teams such as sports; dance; or outdoor activities like biking or hiking. These activities help your child develop balance, motor planning, strength, hand-eye coordination, and confidence in how to move their bodies.

In adolescence, the benefits continue. Physical activity in adolescence can contribute to the development of healthy adult lifestyles, which helps to reduce the chance that a person will have a chronic disease. This can include lower rates of heart disease, diabetes, cancer, and osteoporosis.

Throughout childhood, physical activity—particularly organized sports or activities such as dance, baseball, soccer, or martial arts—provides a regular way to practice impulse control, develop social skills (because to be a good team player you need to think about what your teammates are doing and how you should respond), and have adult role models who go beyond family members.

Healthy physical activity has also been linked to better mood, healthier food choices, more energy during the day, and better sleep quality. Is there anything this magical movement can't do?

There are a few risks to be aware of in promoting physical activity with your kids. Kids who are forced to exercise in childhood and adolescence may reject these activities as adults, leading to them becoming more sedentary. Finding ways to make these activities fun and giving your child choices in activities are key to avoiding this feeling that you are "making them exercise." (See the following Media Can Promote Physical Activity or Displace It section for ways to use media and technology to make physical activity fun for youth.) Early sports specialization is another area to be careful of. Some research studies suggest that kids who specialize in a particular sport early, called *sports specialization*, may have risks of injury or risks of getting burned out and dropping out of the sport. A review article published in the *Journal of Athletic Training* in 2019 showed that injury, overuse injury, serious injuries, and lower extremity injuries were more common in youth with sports specialization. Finding ways that kids enjoy body movement and physical activity, with early exposure to a lot of options for this, seems to be the best approach.

Media Can Promote Physical Activity or Displace It

Different types of media may enhance physical activity or may displace or reduce it. We are not arguing that your child should be physically active every moment they are using media, but a little creativity and activity can be fun for your child. It is OK if your child enjoys media that is more of the sedentary type, but we often don't think of the following ways media use and physical activity can be combined.

Music

Music has a way of getting any of us to move: A great beat, a thumping bass, or a fast tempo can get us tapping our feet or bobbing our heads (Table 6.1). Music can also help us keep moving when we exercise. A 2020 research study published in the journal *Sports* found that listening to music improved running performance.

Table 6.1 | **Ways Music Promotes Movement**

Situation	*How Music Can Be Integrated*
Cleaning up toys, rooms, or your house	Put on music and clean to the beat. Have a challenge to see how many toys can be put away during a particular song. Hold a dance contest with a broom, mop, or vacuum.
Cooking or baking	Put on music and talk about the song or band while you cook with your kids. Stir to the beat (pun intended). Share stories about times you remember hearing a particular favorite song.
After-dinner dance	Have a dance party! Each family member gets to pick one song, and the whole family dances after dinner. When my (Megan) kids were young, we used to do this during Midwest winter nights when we were getting cabin fever. We even bought cheap dance lights and little disco balls to make it cheesier.

Continued on next page

Table 6.1 (*continued*)

Situation	*How Music Can Be Integrated*
Conductor time	Consider acting as conductors in the symphony if your kids enjoy symphonies or classical music. Find some sticks, and proudly direct your own imaginary orchestra through a dramatic classical piece. I (Megan) recommend Beethoven if you want dramatic music with crashing cymbals and Mozart if you want something light, fast-paced, and fun.
Family band night	Allow your kids to choose, make, or find their own instrument. This could include a pot to use as a drum, a kazoo or recorder if your child has one, a play guitar, or actual instruments. Put on a favorite song, and all play along—and get ready for some noise!

Videos

The first type of video that promotes movement is one that focuses on leading you through or teaching you a type of exercise or body movement. These could include workout videos of all sorts—sports training videos; dance videos; stretching videos; and videos that teach yoga, Pilates, or similar types of body movement (Table 6.2). These types of videos don't appeal to every kid (or every adult) but can be a fun way to try a new type of exercise, dance, or body movement before committing to it at school or in a class. These videos can also be something to try together, as your child may be more willing to try something new in a yoga class with you if you are the only two in the class. I (Megan) once had a patient whose mom was trying to get in shape. She was embarrassed to go to a group exercise class but felt unmotivated to exercise alone. She convinced her teen daughter to do dance videos together twice a week in the evening from a streaming platform in their basement. The mom shared how much she appreciated her daughter's support and time, even though she was worried her daughter would think it was "kind of uncool." The daughter smiled quietly and shook her head as mom was talking. When the patient was alone with me, she said, "What my mom doesn't know is that it is really fun for me too."

To enjoy exercising with videos, you'll need to think about where this can happen. If you live in a smaller home or apartment, you may need to think creatively. Can the couches be pushed back to make room in front of the TV? Is there a garage or basement where you can set up a laptop to stream videos? Does your apartment have a deck big enough to do some stretching? Is your yard private enough for a dance session?

Practical Takeaway | **Helping Kids With Coordination Challenges**

Children with developmental coordination challenges or low muscle tone may find sports frustrating and exhausting. It may take them much more effort to kick or throw a ball, perform dance moves, or jog in gym class. Children with hyperflexible joints may ache more after exercising because of misalignment. For these kids, it's important not to avoid physical activity (Jenny has many patients with coordination challenges who would much rather be cozy on a couch with an iPad than on a sports team).

Instead, ask their pediatrician for a referral for occupational therapy (OT) or physical therapy (PT)—this helps with building muscle tone, stamina, and complex motor coordination that kids need for doing a swimming crawl stroke or riding a two-wheeler. OT and PT are usually fun, too, so kids don't mind going.

At home, consider whether there are ways technology can support their exercises. Playing a favorite song or listening to an audio story may help your child engage with these activities.

Table 6.2 | **Videos That Promote Movement**

Type of Video	*How to Use These Videos*
High energy	This category includes dance or concert videos (dance along with performers), as well as aerobic or high-energy cardio videos. Options can range from 10 minutes to sessions lasting more than an hour. Typically, these exercise routines do not require equipment but only space to move. You can consider having a jump rope, an exercise bicycle, or a stepper available to use while watching high-energy videos as another way to enjoy movement. This category is great for older kids or teens who are looking to get in a good workout or relieve stressors through high-energy movement. Younger kids with the wiggles may also benefit from a brief high-energy video.

Continued on next page

Table 6.2 (*continued*)

Type of Video	*How to Use These Videos*
Medium energy	This category includes lower-impact dance or cardio videos, appropriate for all ages. Some videos also provide fitness challenges for younger kids that can incorporate games and pretend, such as pretending to walk or dance like different animals. This category can also include strength training videos that are more appropriate for older kids or teens. If you do not have exercise weights, you can use heavy objects in your house like soup cans or large books. I (Megan) once had a patient whose dad worked in construction use a 2-hold concrete block for weight training, which was great, as long as he was careful to avoid dropping it on his toes.
Low impact	There is an entire range of online exercise videos labeled as "low-energy" workouts, which include low-impact, walk-at-home, or seated workouts and gentle stretching. These videos are appropriate for all ages and can be more accessible for youth or adults with physical challenges or disabilities. Low-impact movement videos also include mind-body practices focused on flexibility, balance, strength, and endurance. These include yoga and Pilates. Routines focused on balance and flexibility also include tai chi and stretching videos. There are even videos designed to introduce young children to yoga through brief routines, as well as videos to engage older children and teens longer term through following a particular creator.
Sports focused	Youth can learn a new sport by finding videos focused on beginners and using step-by-step tutorials. There are also more basic sports-related videos that can build skills such as dribbling a basketball or swinging a tennis racket. If possible, have related sports equipment available to use while watching these videos, and clear out any nearby breakables. These videos focus on learning and may be great for younger children looking to build skills or understand a sport. For older kids or teens, or youth very interested in a particular sport, youth can also practice sports skills with sports performance training videos. The nice thing about these videos is that they build offline skills. Kids might find it easier to transition away from this type of video to go run outside and use their skills on the court or field.

For kids who enjoy videos about physical activity, it may be helpful to identify whether there is a specific channel or creator they can lean into. YouTube has many different channels focused on types of exercise, and following creators who share content that is supportive and engaging may be a great option if your child likes to move with videos. For kids who have physical disabilities, YouTube offers a wealth of videos focused on exercise for kids with physical or mobility challenges.

Be Aware of Negative Content

Keep in mind there is always content out there, particularly online, that promotes unsafe body movement. Think pushing for unreasonable bench presses or 3-hour dance marathons without water or rest. Creators may also use foul or aggressive language in an effort to motivate the viewer. It is a good idea to stay in the loop on whom your child is following and what they are watching online. Consider doing classes together, as it can show your child you are supportive of what they are doing. Yes, this can feel intimidating if you have not been regularly exercising or struggle with physical activity. In this situation, you and your child could select a lower-impact or lower-intensity video for that session. However, your involvement can show that physical activity is something important and something to prioritize and keep working for throughout your life even when it is hard. Our hope is that doing these classes together *can* be fun. Many videos show ways to adapt the activities, such as doing them from a chair or couch or doing mini squats instead of full-on squats. Don't take it too seriously, and move as best you can. If you or your partner is very athletic or enjoys being competitive when exercising, avoid trying to outperform your child. It is not a competition. The goal is to enjoy time together, support moving your bodies for health, and feel connected while doing so.

Video Games

Video games are truly a double-edged sword when it comes to physical activity and kids. Video games can be immersive, exciting, and engaging and can fuel competition and collaboration for your child. Many video games are sedentary—think adventure video games, problem-solving video games, or battle video games. These games may be so immersive that your child sits for way longer than they anticipated when they initially sat down to play.

However, video games or virtual reality (VR) games can also promote physical activity, such as games that allow players to play sports (tennis, golf, soccer), fitness-focused games, or games that center on dancing. These games can be incredible motivators for kids because competitive parts of the game get them to dance faster or harder. These games can also be incredible resources for kids who live in places where outdoor activities are less available or less safe.

Some games offer the opportunity for kids to get outside and be engaged in their environment. One specific example is *Pokémon Go*. A 2016 research study looked at players in *Pokémon Go* and found that over a month of playing it, they increased their activity by more than 1,000 steps a day! They estimated that, overall, *Pokémon Go* added a total of 144 billion steps to physical activity in the United States alone.

TV and Movies

Watching TV and movies (in the theater or at home) is typically thought to be a sedentary activity. Although you can watch videos on your TV, watching TV shows and movies typically doesn't contribute much to body movement. Studies from the pre-smartphone era found that children who watched more than 2 hours a day of TV, or had a TV in their bedroom, were more at risk for being physically inactive. In some cases, these children were also at risk for increased weight, body inflammation, or high blood pressure. The reason for this increased risk was thought to be a combination of inactivity and the risk of eating more while in front of the screen.

Children's TV programming in the past few decades has focused more on getting kids to move their bodies while they watch. Some shows encourage children to mimic the activity the character is doing, such as by

"My neighborhood is not safe. How can I still get movement in during my day?"

This is a common obstacle for families and an area in which media may be helpful in promoting physical activity. Here are some ideas to keep you and your kids moving.

- Try a workout video or DVD (thrift stores have a lot of inexpensive workout and dance DVDs).
- See if there is a location near home or school that is safe and promotes activity, such as a YMCA, Boys & Girls Club, or community recreation center.
- Consider video games that promote activity such as sports, dance, or other movement skills.

Practical Takeaway | **"But I don't have time for physical activity!"**

Many kids are busy these days, going to school, doing homework, engaging in activities, doing chores, or working after school. Parents may want their children to be physically active but know they have limited time. Adding some movement into their already scheduled media time is an effective way to incorporate some physical activity into an activity your child already enjoys on a regular basis.

jumping or running in place. *Dora the Explorer* is a show that encourages kids to hop, skip, and jump along with the characters at certain points in the episode.

Outdoor Physical Activity

It can be tricky to talk about integrating technology into outdoor physical activity, as many people have strong beliefs about what is or is not appropriate in outdoor recreation. We are not suggesting that everyone benefits from including technology in the great outdoors. However, there is nothing inherently wrong with incorporating technology into your experience as long as it follows a couple simple rules.

- The technology should be present to enhance the existing outdoor experience, not distract from it.
- The technology should not distract from anyone else's outdoor experience.

A major way to avoid distracting others is by avoiding technology that reaches other people's senses, such as their sight or hearing. Technology with flashing lights or bright lights that are distracting to others can be distracting from the beauty of the outdoors, whether it is day or night. Technology that makes noise that others can hear, including playing music on small speakers, can interfere with others' enjoyment of being outside. Dim your brights and wear headphones.

A Favorite Patient Story From Megan

Mika (patient's name has been changed) is a 15-year-old born into a family of avid hikers who believe that being outdoors is an antidote to modern life. However, Mika is really into creating music using different apps, reading books, and baking. She grumbles her way through weekend hikes with her dad, enjoying his excitement but not really sharing it. During hikes, the one thing she does show interest in is asking about the different flowers and plants. However, her dad usually can't remember what they are. Each year, her dad and uncle plan a hiking and camping trip for Mika and her cousins. This year, her dad really wants her to enjoy the trip. He thinks about how to find ways to make the trip feel interesting to her. He downloads an app that lets him identify local flowers and trees, as well as a stargazing app. On the hiking trail, when Mika asks about a flower, he shows her the app, and they look it up together. Mika is excited and starts to look for new flowers and trees as they hike the trail. That evening at the campfire, Mika and her cousins take turns using the stargazing app to identify different constellations. Mika loves that her dad was able to find ways to make sure she enjoyed the trip by merging her interests along with his.

Promoting Physical Activity in Your Family

Busy families need plans to make things happen, including physical activity. Look at your family calendar or calendars to see where activities could fit in. Do you have any of the following?

- Ten minutes in the morning while the coffee brews to do a quick video together
- Opportunity to walk your kids to a common destination (school, park, library) on a regular basis
- Time to do a bike ride on the weekends
- A break before or after dinner to schedule in 30 minutes of body movement

In addition to considering technology to support body movement, you can use technology to schedule activity so that it is on your online calendar. If you have a paper calendar, write down your planned physical activity, and consider adding stickers or stars on the days you are successful. If your family uses an online calendar, track it there and add smiley faces or bright colors to the entry to celebrate each accomplishment.

Key Point

How much physical activity does your child need?

The American Academy of Pediatrics recommends at least 60 minutes of moderate to vigorous physical activity daily for kids aged 6 to 17. Younger kids need active play throughout the day, with a focus on fun and variety.

If You Are Worried That Media Is Displacing Your Child's Physical Activity

If you are worried about media and technology displacing your child from getting a healthy amount of physical activity, it is important to take steps to understand the issue, create possible solutions, implement a plan, and monitor the outcomes.

You may be concerned because you notice your child spending excessive time using media such as watching screens or playing games. You may have noticed your child is less active and more sedentary. This situation suggests that media may be displacing time that could be spent on physical activity. You might also notice that after your child engages with media they have lost motivation to engage in physical activity, which they might perceive as "too hard" after the fun of shows or video games. I (Jenny) have sometimes found that children with weaker *proprioception* (the sense of where your body is in space) almost lose track of their body's signals when they are immersed in a video game. They might need a few of what OTs call "grounding" or "organizing" activities that help them pay attention to their body's signals, such as the sensory input their arms, legs, and skin are feeling.

To understand the issue better, you need additional information from your child about their use of technology.

Research Corner | **Motivators for Physical Activity**

One 2012 research study looked at how teens used technology to engage in physical activity. I (Megan) was a mentor on this research published in the *ISRN Obesity* journal. We conducted focus groups with both younger teens (ages 12–15) and older teens (ages 16–18). We learned that younger teens often described technology as a complement to physical activity. One study participant shared, "We're just running around, and there's nothing to listen to, but when there is music on, everyone feels like, oh, this is fun, let's run around, let's be fun."

Older teens described technology as a motivator for physical activity. One example was seeing social media posts from friends describing going for a run or learning a new gymnastics skill, and this would motivate them to also do these activities.

We also learned that teens' views of technology and physical activity differed by community type. Adolescents in rural settings often described being outdoors for exercise. One participant shared, "I walk around our property and walk my dog." But adolescents living in urban settings often described indoor activities. One participant stated, "I've got workout videos, like DVDs, and I go to the gym." Another participant described using a gaming system and shared, "That's definitely for fitness because everything you do is moving like your shoulders and stuff...it really gets you moving 'cause you really get into it." This study was one of the first to show ways that teens used technology for physical activity that differed by age and community type. It also showed how creative teens can be in using technology in healthy ways.

How are they spending their time? This question can help you understand if there are other stressors or activities that they are worried about or are using media to escape from or whether they are bored and need more activities to fill their time.

What are they watching or playing? This question can help you understand more about their media use, as well as whether there are opportunities to incorporate more activity during their media use.

How do they feel during, or after, they use media? This question can help your child build on their own reflections about how they feel. Do they feel exhausted and drained after a 2-hour TV marathon? Did they use media to calm down but now feel more anxious? Linking these feelings to how they'd like to approach their media differently can be a powerful way to help them build reflection skills and connections between behaviors and feelings.

You'll also want to know about their physical activity and how they are feeling about their current level of activity. If your child is pretty inactive but doesn't think it is an issue, you may need to have some conversations about the health benefits of physical activity outlined at the start of this chapter.

Once you understand how your child is spending their time, and how they are feeling about it, you can create possible solutions. Depending on your child's age, try to find ways to include them in coming up with solutions and setting concrete goals. Some example goals could include adding in 30 minutes of physical activity daily, with a concrete plan for what type of activity, when it will happen, and how parents can check in that this is happening.

Once the plan is in place, it is important to monitor and find ways to celebrate your child's success. Let them know you've noticed them working hard and keeping up with their outlined goals. Particularly in the first days of starting the new routine, try to catch them being good and provide positive feedback and reinforcement. There may be some slipups or setbacks, and it is important to also recognize those setbacks and encourage your child on how to get back on track. If you do implement consequences for not following the plan, such as limitations on technology use, be sure to stick with what you said would happen. If you plan to have consequences for not following the plan and you do not follow through, it teaches your child that your consequences are not real.

Anxiety + Technology

I (Megan) once had a patient referred to me for concerns about excessive video game use. This patient was in a bad place emotionally with school stress and a recent breakup with a long-term girlfriend. He had been a star baseball player but quit the team. He would go online to game with friends late into the night, after his parents were in bed, so at first, they were unaware this was occurring. They realized how much their child was gaming once his grades started to slip, and they learned he had quit baseball. His parents tried to set limits by shutting off the Wi-Fi at 10 pm, but their child threatened to go live with an aunt. The parents felt at their wit's end.

This was a very tough situation that involved starting with the patient's mental health and realizing he had symptoms of anxiety that had not been addressed. Video games were a temporary solution he used to manage his anxiety and stress, but it was clearly not a good long-term healthy approach.

A referral to a counselor was an initial step. We also talked about the role of physical activity in managing symptoms. He started with short-distance runs 2 days a week to get back in shape. Working with the patient and his parents, we set limits on his gaming at night to ensure he got enough sleep, with a stop time of 10 pm, which was an initial goal given his previous bedtime was 2 am. We discussed the importance of his physical and mental health and how that could be supported through physical activity and sleep. It took months for him to get back to a place where he really felt healthy.

There was progress made in the first couple months, then a backslide for a few weeks, then a renewed commitment from the patient that lasted 6 months, and then a tough period including refusal to engage in treatment for a full month. But things eventually improved, and the patient later shared that the emphasis on what he should do to be healthy, including being active and getting sleep, helped him focus on what to *do* with his time rather than what *not* to do (play video games all night).

Connecting the Dots

Embodied experiences like playing, dancing, outdoor activities, and sports are a crucial part of human well-being. Carving out the time for these experiences on a daily basis is difficult for busy families, so work with your kids to create regular movement routines—and also find spontaneous moments. We can't recommend dance parties enough as a way to combine media, social connection, and getting energy out.

- **Engage in a challenge:** If starting a physical activity routine is newer for your child or your family, do a challenge to start low and go slow. Many kids, especially teens, who have been sedentary will want to jump into rigorous or sustained exercise right away. This aggressive approach can often lead to kids feeling sore, tired, or frustrated and calling the whole thing off. Try a challenge to move your bodies consistently for a month. Start with 5 minutes a day together for a week, maybe stretching or walking. Add some fun music, listen to an audiobook or podcast, or watch a stretching video. Then try for 10 minutes daily in week 2, 15 in week 3, and 20 in week 4, maybe using some videos that show dances or exercises you enjoy. Then sit with your child and decide where you want to go for month 2. This low and slow approach is more likely to be sustained, and doable, for families who are newer to moving their bodies.
- **Talk to your friends:** How do they integrate media into their physical activity? Or don't they? It can be easy to get stuck in a routine or feel stuck in a rut when it comes to physical activity, but friends can be a great source of genius ideas.

Chapter 7

DIET AND NUTRITION

What we will cover

- A few reminders about nutrition's role in supporting your child's growth
- Exploring different ways that nutrition shows up across various types of media
- How you can make sure that media is not your child's only teacher regarding nutrition

Nutrition is not an easy topic to cover in a book about media, as the topic is so big, and parents bring so much expertise to the table in navigating how to feed their children. Nutrition has ties to family traditions, cultural importance, evidence-based guidelines, and child preferences. These days, nutrition also has ties to "what I eat in a day" videos, perfectly curated "mascarpone-topped tarte tatin" posted photos, and food influencers on social media. On top of that, children's eating patterns and preferences change as they grow, so it can feel like hitting a moving target, especially if you have more than one child to feed. Any parent who has had their child go through the "I only eat white foods," or "I'd rather die than eat broccoli," or "I read that I should be on a low-carb diet so no more bread," phase, knows how tough this topic can be when raising children. The good news about nutrition is that there are a lot of strategies in how to approach feeding your kids no matter what their preferences are.

Nutrition's Role in Child Growth and Development

As every parent knows, nutrition is critical to your child's growth and development. Throughout childhood, nutrition provides the fuel for playing, learning, growing, laughing, crying, and everything in between. At its most simple, nutrition needs to provide energy to fuel the body, and it needs to provide essential nutrients to allow key functions of our physical bodies to work well. Nutrient deficiencies, such as a lack of vitamin C or not enough protein in the diet, can limit growth, harm our immune systems, slow development, and increase the risk of illness.

Where Does Nutrition Show Up in Media?

Media provides a great deal of teaching and role modeling about nutrition, but like any other topic on the internet, it can share inaccurate health information or norms you don't agree with. This is why it is important for parents to understand what messages media teaches so that they can ensure that media is not the *only* teacher on this topic. For this section, we walk through different types of media and common ways that those media outlets teach about nutrition. We'll mention the common age ranges affected and the most frequent types of messages.

How Does Media Influence Diet and Nutrition?

There are a couple ways that media can influence our choices and opinions about what we eat. One explanation is that seeing food in the media leads us to think that that food is normal and what other people eat, so we should eat it too. This is often referred to as *establishing social norms* or *social influence theory.*

Another explanation is that we learn specific steps about *how* to do behaviors from social media. The *social learning theory* argues that media is a powerful teacher of specifics about how to do things. It argues that you can learn to fix a broken pipe by watching an online video that shows someone doing the step-by-step instructions; if you do exactly what they

Research Corner | **The 2-Group Experiment**

Many of the studies shared in this chapter feature a common approach found in several research studies involving 2 groups for comparison. In the experiment, each group watches different content in media; one group watches content that is food related, and the other watches content unrelated to food. Or one group is exposed to food that has low nutritional value, such as sweets or fast food, and the other group sees food that is high in nutritional value such as fruits and vegetables. After this exposure to media, the researchers observe behavior, such as what kinds of food the research participants select from a buffet or how much they eat.

As an example, in one study from the journal *Appetite,* researchers asked one group of participants to watch a cooking show and the other group to watch a nature show. After the viewings, both groups were presented with 800 total calories of sweets (chocolate and candy), salty snacks (cheese curls), and carrots. The group who watched the cooking show ate significantly more sweets than the group who watched the nature show did. This study design can show the kinds of influences the media has on people's food choices and behaviors in the short term.

do, you will fix the pipe. This theory supports the idea that when we watch other people eat certain foods and show how to make them, we want to do those same steps because we have now learned how.

A 2020 study from the journal *Appetite* tested these theories in the world of social media. The investigators found that people generally viewed what they saw on a social media site as "normal" and adjusted their eating habits to be similar to those of the people they saw on social media. The results of this study may be a combination of both social influence theory and social learning theory, and they show how powerful the influence of social media can be on our own behavior.

Media representations of food can also prime us. Seeing food can activate our hunger and our brain regions for reward, creating a desire for that food. Exposure to appetizing food can trigger feelings of hunger, even if we were not hungry before we viewed that content.

Definitions

Social influence theory: This theory supports the idea that people want to follow what others do in order to be accepted, so if they see that many or most people are doing a particular behavior, they want to do it too. Social influence is a powerful tool for why we want to do certain things to fit in with others.

Social learning theory: This theory illustrates the human drive to learn from others. It argues that if we want to learn to do something new, we can learn how to do it by watching someone else do it (ideally someone who knows what they are doing).

Finally, social media provides us with a sense of reinforcement of what is good. If we see an influencer or gamer or celebrity eating a certain food, and that person gets positive feedback for that behavior from likes and comments, it makes it seem like the behavior is rewarding. If a food-based social media post gets a lot of likes, we may interpret this as that the food is good.

These influences may affect us differently in different situations and can influence us in ways that are conscious or subconscious. In a 2009 study from the journal *Health Psychology*, the authors tested priming effects of TV food advertising on eating behavior. Researchers did 2 experiments. In the experiment with an adult population, they showed participants food advertisements and then offered food to eat, and those who ate more food after seeing the advertisements *insisted* that they were not affected by the advertisements. Furthermore, the amount of food consumed after watching the advertisements did not relate to the participants' reported hunger, so they ate food and snacks regardless of whether they were hungry at the time. This study suggested that food-related ads and content tap into our *fast-brain* responses—our implicit (not *slow-brain* thoughtful and contemplative) ways to react to stimuli. (See page 152 for results of the second experiment.) Technology platforms also use these fast-brain responses. On any platform that collects data about users (eg, social media, online games, AI chatbots), we can be profiled based on what stimuli we react to and then sent more persuasive ads about those things. In other words, if you click on or hover over content with energy drinks, you'll get more ads for energy drinks.

Food Commercials

There have been decades of research on how effective commercials are designed and placed to reach and influence kids. If you grew up in the days of Saturday morning cartoons on TV, you probably remember the numerous commercials for cereal. These commercials were designed to reach kids and appeal to their sugar cravings. They had colorful and cheerful designs to attract kids' attention, get them excited about the cereal (and maybe a toy in the box), and provide prompts to ask their parents for that cereal. This phenomenon of kids bugging their parents to buy a particular type of food or snack was so powerful and common that it was referred to by marketers as *pester power*.

Fast food is another area in which food commercials have been (and continue to be) very effective. These commercials were also typically designed to capture the attention of children. If you ever question whether kids really pay attention to fast-food commercials, keep in mind this study from the *Archives of Pediatrics & Adolescent Medicine* in 2007 in which the researchers presented 3- to 5-year-olds with 5 types of food. They were offered the food in plain wrapping or in McDonald's wrapping. The researchers found that the children preferred the food they thought was from McDonald's compared with the same food in plain wrapping. In this study, children as young as 3 years old could recognize the McDonald's brand, associate it with Ronald McDonald, and state clear preferences for food with that branding. Remarkably, 2 of the 5 foods that the children were presented with were baby carrots and milk, and even then, the children still described that they liked the food more when it was presented in McDonald's packaging. Cartoon characters such as Ronald McDonald are a common way that food marketers capture the attention and adoration of kids. They develop a friendly character that they can use to catch children's attention to help sell more food. Think of the gr-r-reat effect that Tony the Tiger has had on selling Kellogg's Frosted Flakes since their creation.

Movies

You may think that movies are free of nutritional content, as usually there are no ads and the focus is on the story, but keep in mind that movies are actually huge educators in the topic of nutrition. Movies can include iconic characters who love a particular type of food that becomes a large part of the story. My (Megan) kids loved the Wallace and Gromit movies when they were young and would yell out "Cheeeese, Gromit!" at random intervals whenever we had meals with cheese included.

Another approach that movies use is having a company pay for product placement in various movie scenes. One example is an old but famous movie—*E. T. the Extra-Terrestrial.* The prominent showing of E.T.'s love of Reese's Pieces provided incredible revenue for that company because of that specific product placement. A 1998 study in the *Journal of Current Issues & Research in Advertising* studied product placements in movies and revealed that in the 3 months immediately after *E. T.*'s release, sales of Reese's Pieces increased by 65%.

Research Corner | **Advertising Exposure**

In one research study from 2024 published in *JAMA Network Open,* the study team examined US advertising exposure for young children (2- to 5-year-olds) and school-age children (6- to 11-year-olds) between 2013 and 2022. The researchers studied trends over time in advertisements for foods low in nutritional value, such as fast food and sweets. Although they found some decreases in the percentages of advertisements for these low-nutritional–value foods over the decade, the percentages of advertisements were still quite high. In children's programming for ages 2 to 5, about 64% of advertisements were for low-nutritional–value foods. For children's programming for 6- to 11-year-olds, about 60% of all advertisements were for low-nutritional–value foods. Even where advertisements decreased over time, the most common type of advertisements during children's programming still featured low-nutritional–value foods.

Research Corner | **Product Placement in Movies**

A 2010 study published in the journal *Pediatrics* reviewed food and beverage brand placements in a large sample of popular movies between 1996 and 2005. Of the 200 movies they examined, 69% included one food, beverage, or food retail establishment brand. The most common types of food were candy and sweets (26%), salty snacks (21%), and sugar-sweetened beverages like soda (76%). Of the food retail establishments included in movies, two-thirds were fast-food restaurants.

Does product placement in movies really influence your child? After all, it is not an advertisement, so it is not overtly selling something, right? Does it really influence food preferences and behavior?

One study in 2004 from the *Journal of Consumer Research* used the 2-group model of dividing children into 2 groups for exposure to media. Both groups saw a brief film clip from the movie *Home Alone*. One group saw the actual film clip, which showed the beverage Pepsi being spilled during a meal. The other group saw a similar clip, but the brand name was removed from the soda bottle. After the movie clip, all participants were invited to help themselves to Pepsi or Coca-Cola at the start of a research interview. Children who saw the unbranded version of the movie clip picked Pepsi or Coke with relatively similar frequency. Children who saw the Pepsi version of the movie clip chose Pepsi over Coke almost twice as often.

Finally, sometimes the focus of the movie is on food itself. Think of *Big Night*, *Julie & Julia*, or even *Ratatouille*. The approach of a story about food is not universally a negative thing. It depends on the story of the movie and what is being taught about nutrition or the role of food in families and culture. In some cases, these storylines can help children understand that making good food is not always easy to do but that the effort can be rewarding. Some of these stories focus on how food and meals can bring people together and foster great conversations. Other movies may focus on food in less healthy ways, such as themes around body image, eating disorders (more on this topic in Chapter 12), or overconsumption of unhealthy foods. Stories are powerful teachers, and movies are an investment of time and interest. When those stories involve food, they share what is normal or what is possible, as well as different ways to view food.

Movie Tie-Ins

Another strategy is tying a food product to a big blockbuster movie. Think of fast-food restaurants doing a campaign for a new children's movie, with specially branded cups or limited time giveaways. These campaigns can attract fans of the movie or characters and lead them to want to go to the restaurant more to collect all the movie-related stuff they can.

Video Games and Game Apps

Video games are another place where food-related content shows up in more ways than you might initially think. Some of the most iconic video games are about eating. A classic example is *Pac-Man*, where the little chomping icon has to eat as many pellets and fruits as possible. Or *Burger Time,* in which you walk over (that doesn't seem like it would meet food safety standards) parts of a burger to have them come together in a stack.

As with any type of content, there are some video games that many may view as containing problematic messages. *Fat Princess* is one in which players feed cake to a princess who gradually gains weight making it more difficult to carry her to the castle. Roblox has a popular game called *Fat Simulator* in which the goal is to eat as much as possible and grow bigger than the other players. Bodies and food can be used as *clickbait*—types of content and images that compel us to click—and is a large reason why they get used as attention-grabbing designs in video games.

Video Game Advertisements

You may be thinking, well, at least there is no marketing or advertising of foods in video games. But there is. Ads also frequently pop up in children's mobile apps. Another approach is through *video game live streaming platforms.*

Definition

What is a **video game live streaming platform**? These platforms are social networks for gamers. Users can broadcast or watch video game footage as it happens via live stream. They can also communicate with other users while it happens. These platforms can be accessed by computer, tablet, smartphone, and some gaming consoles.

One popular platform shows a main video stream of the current game in action as well as the gamer (also called a *gaming influencer*). Below this main screen is the stream title, and there is a side screen with a live chat.

Live streaming platforms feature advertisements, and in 2024 a group of researchers published a study in the journal *Appetite*. The researchers analyzed the food cues on Twitch, a popular video game live streaming platform, by influencers likely to be popular with adolescents. They found that the most common food advertisements were for energy drinks, such as Red Bull or Monster Energy, and fast food. These can show up as advertisements or be promoted directly by influencers eating and drinking particular products while they are gaming. A unique aspect of this marketing is that users are watching the influencer/gamer enjoy the food in real time, which may be influential for teens to feel like they are part of that moment and copy what the gamer is doing.

Real-Time Product Placement

Monster Energy drinks has a yearly promotional event with the *Call of Duty* video game. The promotion has a unique code for gamers to unlock bonus content and rewards. You can see why both companies benefit, as more energy drink consumption keeps gamers playing longer.

Video Game Product Placement

Food products have also paid money to be included in video games. For example, Doritos chips had a custom Doritos chip emote on a video game streaming platform. An energy drink was branded as the Official Energy Drink of Esports.

Definition

Esports, or **electronic sports,** are organized, competitive video games. In these tournaments, individuals and teams who play video games professionally engage in play for prizes, product endorsements, entertainment, and money. These tournaments have grown in popularity and are often streamed online to viewers.

There are also some games that may provide a glimpse of real-life experiences. *Diner Dash* is a game in which the player runs a diner and must serve all the customers, sometimes even cooking the food. This game may shed some light on the challenges of running a restaurant. There are several game apps that also center on making food, such as *Toca Kitchen*, or the challenges of running a food-related business, such as *Travellers Rest*. Unfortunately, there is not yet a lot of research on the effect of these types of experiential games, although it has been suggested that they can expose children who are picky or curious eaters to different food combinations.

Practical Takeaway | Know Your Media

Wondering if that new game your child is asking for has problematic food content? Common Sense Media has an entire page (www.commonsensemedia.org/parents-ultimate-guides/gaming) focused on reviewing these games and is a great resource for you and your kids to use before a game is purchased or downloaded.

Social Media

Social media includes advertisements and influencers, and both have significant influence on nutrition. The different types of social media trends and their pros and cons are outlined in Table 7.1.

In addition to highly stylized professional ads and influencer content, social media also includes content from a youth's peers and friends. So let's talk about user-generated videos that your child may see and be influenced by. Peers have the ability to create posts, videos, and captions to represent their own experiences. Some trends that show up on social media and influence youth include food photos and videos. Although there are also images and videos out there created by influencers or celebrities, content from someone you know hits home a little differently. Peer content can feel more accessible and influential. A teen may know she can't ever be exactly like her favorite pop star but has better odds at being like her friend down the street.

Table 7.1 | **Food Trends on Social Media**

Social Media Trend	*Pros and Cons*
Taking photos of fancy dishes or plates at restaurants (often referred to as *food porn*)	*Pro:* Can be fun to see these artful photos of fancy food. Creative teens may enjoy staging these photos of dishes at home. *Con:* These dishes are often desserts, which can lead to an overrepresentation of sweet foods. These photos can present food that is high in sugar and low in nutritional value and also can prime the viewer to want food like that. Fancy food photos can also highlight disparities in access to food, showing food that is high in calories as well as cost. These posts can then lead teens and other users who cannot access this type of food to feel "less than."
What I eat in a day (#WIEIAD whatieatinaday)	*Pro:* This trend of food videos has become immensely popular, leading to specific videos for people who are gluten-free or have other dietary restrictions, which can help teens find new, safe dishes to try. *Con:* Some videos include an unhealthy focus on calorie intake, portion sizes, and protein content. Others include unhealthy behaviors, such as *body checking* (see Chapter 12 for more on this). These videos can present a daily intake with unhealthy expectations or promises, leaving a viewer to feel self-conscious or anxious about what they eat. And there are no guarantees about the accuracy of the content, the qualifications of the creator, or the feasibility or accessibility of the viewer being able to create that food.

Continued on next page

Table 7.1 (*continued*)

Social Media Trend	*Pros and Cons*
Mukbang (The word mukbang [meokbang] is a portmanteau of the Korean words for eating [meongneun] and broadcast/show [bangsong], sometimes labeled online as "eating show.")	These videos initially emerged in South Korea with a focus on eating copious amounts of food alone or in groups, usually without talking. The videos were often watched for the sheer enormity of food consumed as entertainment, but some viewers used them as ASMR (see Chapter 5) to relax to the consistent sounds of eating. Nearly a decade later, these videos have shifted over time and adapted to cultures in which they have been popular. The US version of mukbang often focuses on eating food on video that is incredibly messy, like dripping with sauce, or visually appealing with bright colors like ketchup on macaroni and cheese. *Pro:* The current popularity of mukbang focuses more on "normal" amounts of consumed food rather than extreme volumes. *Con:* Some argue that these videos celebrate eating, countering the social media cultural norms of thinness and depriving oneself in order to be thin. Others feel disgusted by watching these videos, either due to the messiness or the volume of food. Some have suggested these videos also highlight the loneliness around the fact that so many people eat alone and film themselves.

How social media images shape norms

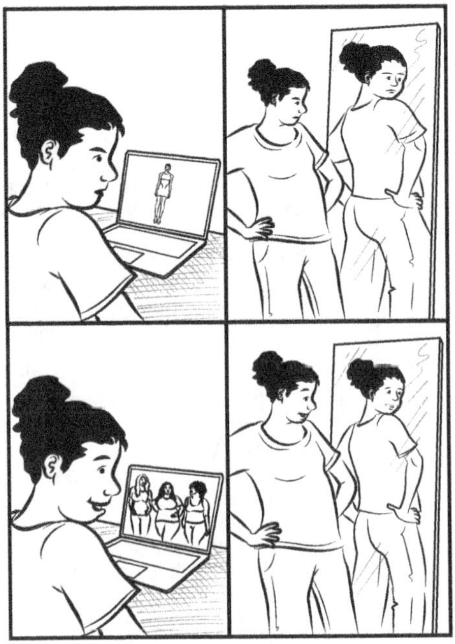

Celebrity Endorsements and Influencers

Another approach to nutrition is through celebrity endorsements, which can show up on TV, in movies or commercials, or in social media posts. One campaign that really showcased the power of celebrity influencers was the Got Milk? campaign that launched in California in the 1990s. The campaign is credited with saving the then-faltering California dairy industry from an estimated $200 million in annual losses due to declining sales. This single campaign was reported to have achieved more than 90% brand awareness and to have made milk cool again through its wide array of celebrity spokespeople. The campaign included an incredible list of celebrities across actors, musicians, and athletes, including Beyoncé, Shaquille O'Neal, Taylor Swift, Danica Patrick, Naomi Campbell, and even the Muppets.

Influencers of today are a little different but with some similarities. These can include those with wide reach and appeal, such as lifestyle influencers who may promote fashion, cars, and other products alongside nutritional products. One popular approach is identifying lifestyle influencers to promote specific products such as brands of water, energy drinks, snacks, or soda. Other influencers focus solely on nutrition. These influencers can include actual dieticians, as well as health and wellness personalities. These influencers may share recipes, meal prep ideas, and health tips, but at the end of the day, they are usually still doing this in order to sell products.

The risk of nutrition-focused influencers is that, despite their background or expertise, some influencers' goals are not education or accuracy but rather generating engagement and selling products. A 2023 news story illustrated an issue that arose when a group of nutrition influencers shared inaccurate information about aspartame and other artificial sweeteners. This group shared posts on social media promoting these products as safe, and they shared information that conflicted with warnings about the safety of these products as "possibly carcinogenic" but within acceptable intake limits from the World Health Organization. The Federal Trade Commission issued warnings to these influencers and found that food industry trade groups were paying these influencers to share this information via social media. In late 2025, the Federal Trade Commission released a report, *Disclosures 101 for Social Media Influencers*, that specified that influencers must comply with the law when making recommendations about products; if influencers don't disclose a financial relationship to the product and brand, the law sees this as deceptive marketing.

A 2020 study in the *International Journal of Environmental Research and Public Health* invited children aged 10 to 11 to watch a social media video showing influencer marketing and discuss their thoughts. A key theme from the study was that children felt they connected to influencers as aspirational and familiar role models. This familiarity meant that social media influencers had a greater effect because they were known to the child. Even at younger ages, youth recognize the role that influencers can play in affecting their preferences and behaviors. This article was titled "It's Just Addictive People That Make Addictive Videos" to represent the views of the participants.

Why Do Unhealthy Foods Get So Much Attention?

Nutrition scientists have developed a list called the *Big Five* to describe types of foods that have the combination of a *low* level of nutritional value and a *high* level of calories.

The following are the types of foods that are best to have in moderation or not at all:

- Sweets, candy, chocolate
- Soft drinks and soda
- Salty processed snacks such as chips
- Fast food
- Sugary breakfast cereal

One 2005 research study from the *American Journal of Public Health* found that of all the food commercials shown during TV shows that children watch most, more than 80% were for foods included on the Big Five list. These are the foods that are being shown to kids in commercials and promoted as foods children should be interested in and ask their parents to purchase. This may come as a new realization, or a reminder, but it is important to think about how media, particularly commercials, try to teach your child about nutrition and how they appeal to their attention.

Research has found that YouTubers popular with young children often feature high-pleasure foods such as candy and fast food as an engagement tactic. In one of my (Jenny) studies published in 2024 in *JAMA Network Open*, we analyzed video *thumbnails* (the small snapshots that advertise what will be in a YouTube video) and found heaps of pizza, candy, lollipops, and chocolate bars—sometimes with a huge mouth about to eat them—kind of bizarre! But if you think about it, these high-pleasure items often attract attention from young kids with weaker impulse control, which translates to more ad clicks and more ad dollars for the YouTuber.

For teens, social media viewing patterns can lead to following companies, celebrities, or influencers promoting unhealthy foods or diets. Social media can also trigger pop-up advertisements showing these products or trends. In one of my (Megan) studies in 2012 published in *Cyberpsychology, Behavior, and Social Networking*, we created a social media profile and entered different types of statements about diet and fitness habits as status updates posted to the platform. Examples included healthy patterns such as "best salad ever for lunch" and less healthy statements such as "All I've eaten today is a soda and 3 Pop-Tarts." We then analyzed the pop-up advertisements that appeared once the status update was posted. The pop-up advertisements in response to those posts included about 10% advertising fad diets, including the "Oreo cookie diet," which promotes eating nothing but Oreo cookies. The statement that generated the most diet- and fitness-related advertisements referred to being underweight—"was turned away from giving blood today because I didn't weigh enough ☹"—and led to more than 65% of the advertisements focusing on fitness and diet, including an ad for the "fat-burning furnace," a supplement to promote weight loss. This experiment showed us how social media algorithms deliver targeted, but often very unhealthy, advertisements in response to posting any content about diet or fitness.

Nutritional Supplements

Another area to be aware of as a parent is content that is being delivered to children about nutritional supplements. This may happen via advertisements on TV or social media and via influencers or celebrities. These supplements often follow trends in popularity; some popular ones have included collagen, magnesium, ashwagandha, creatine, and biotin. Although there is evidence for use of some supplements in people with specific conditions, supplements often make promises of benefits that teens find important, such as improving skin or hair or gaining muscle.

Prevention: How to Have Conversations About Nutrition

Eating nutritional foods and learning to enjoy them during childhood is critical to short- and long-term health. Fruits improve heart health, decrease risks of colon cancer, and decrease depression. Increased vegetable intake decreases the risk of colon cancer, hip fracture, stroke, and depression. Food is sustenance, and food is also growth; development; and, in some cases, medicine. The main strategies to make fruits, vegetables, and other nutritious foods appealing to kids include health literacy, as well as good communication and feeding patterns.

Finding Positive Food Marketing and Media Messages

Several research studies have directly looked at how viewing media leads to eating patterns and food choices. Let's talk about the second experiment in that 2009 study from the journal *Health Psychology*. This experiment worked with 2 groups of children. The first group watched a video with advertisements for food, like fast food or sweet cereal. The other group saw a video with advertisements that did not feature food. Then they provided both groups of children with access to a buffet with a variety of food on it. It may not surprise you that the kids who watched the video with food advertisements chose the sweets 45% more than the other group did. This study tells us that it is not just the content of the TV show that influences nutrition choices but also the advertisements.

Practical Takeaway | **Finding Positive Food-Related Content**

One approach that parents can take is to seek out media content that showcases nutritious foods. Common Sense Media has a large library of TV shows you can review to inform choices for your family. They have a specific recommendations section for shows of this type that include shows for younger kids, such as *Sesame Street,* and shows for older kids, like *Jamie Oliver's Food Revolution.* (Note: Parents can access an initial set of reviews for free; after that a paid account is needed).

Evaluate Negative Food Marketing and Media Messages

Encourage your child, through gentle prodding or with questions, to think critically about the presence of food product placement in movies or shows. I (Megan) once had a patient whose father was a senior advertising executive, and he shared that anytime he watched a movie with his kids and saw a food product he would ask his kids to guess how much that company had paid to be in that one movie scene. It became a game, and they would then research the actual cost. It led to many interesting discussions about the lengths that company was willing to go to in order to put a particular food or product in a movie. Similarly, when food appears as clickbait in thumbnails or social media videos, help your children recognize this as an engagement tactic (Table 7.2), and avoid those videos. These discussions can be fun and spirited and can help your child develop the media literacy skills to ask, "What is being sold to me and why?"

Table 7.2 | **Playing Media Literacy Detective**

Situation	*Possible Questions and Prompts*
An influencer shares a social media post drinking a branded type of coffee (or soda or tea)	Do you think that influencer actually likes that coffee? How much would a company need to pay you to advertise something you don't like? Why do you think this post showed up in your feed? Do you think you're more likely to try that coffee because of this post? Why or why not?
A commercial for cereal is featured during a morning show	Why do you think this commercial is showing up now? Who do you think this message is for? What parts of this ad are meant to influence kids? Is the ad effective? What message is this advertisement trying to tell kids?
A commercial for pizza delivery comes on during an afternoon sports game	Why do you think this commercial is showing up now? Who do you think this message is for? What parts of this ad are meant to influence kids? How about parents? Is the ad effective? What message is this advertisement trying to tell kids?

Protect Mealtime

Parents can affect their children's nutrition by protecting mealtimes together such as family dinners. Research studies have found that families that eat dinner together more frequently have more health and well-being benefits from this practice, including healthier nutritional choices, better mental health and well-being, and healthy weight management. One study from 2014 from *JAMA Pediatrics* examined youth who had experienced cyberbullying and found that frequency of family dinners was protective from the negative consequences of bullying. And it is not just youth who benefit. Another study in 2024 from *Maternal & Child Nutrition* found that moms with toddlers had significant mental health benefits linked to frequency of family meals. This study described family meals as a time when child-rearing and nutrition were woven together and showed the power of bringing family members together for food and conversation. Family dinners can allow each member of the family to be heard, to ask questions, or to share something of themselves. It is a way to come together regularly and thus to see that, even when dinners get tense, stressful, quiet, or challenging, the next evening is another chance to come together and be present for each other. Day by day and year by year, these gatherings have incredible power to nourish children's physical and mental health.

Does this mean you need to provide a perfectly balanced 3-course meal for dinner every night of the week? Heck no! The magic of family dinner is that it is a *family* dinner. You are eating together, talking together, and enjoying time and food together. Some nights may include leftovers. Other nights it may be takeout. And, if you're lucky, some nights it might be pancakes. My (Megan) family is known to enjoy breakfast food for dinner. We also occasionally have what we call *Picky-Picky* dinner made up of a collection of snacks, cut-up veggies, and leftovers in homage to the family cat in the Ramona Quimby books by Beverly Cleary. In a Picky-Picky dinner, you can pick a little of this and pick a little of that and try to avoid being too picky like Ramona's cat, who refused cat food but ate part of their jack-o'-lantern. Family meals teach your children to be together and enjoy food together, even if the food is not worthy of a #WIEIAD photo.

Connecting the Dots

Media content about nutrition can be positive, promoting togetherness during meals, encouraging experimentation with cooking, and helping you feel good about nourishing your body. Media content about nutrition can also promote foods that have a lot of calories and very little nutrition or encourage unhealthy eating habits. In a digital world where media constantly markets food to our children, the dinner table becomes more than a place to eat. It becomes a place to teach, question, connect, and model what a healthy relationship with food looks like. Viewing media together to ensure it has a healthy message is critical and can help build lifelong skills and values around nutritious food.

- **Conduct an experiment:** Go to www.youtube.com and search for *Device Free Dinner with Will Ferrell.* When possible, watch the video together as a family. This video was created as part of the Device Free Dinner campaign by Common Sense Media. Released in 2017, it features actor Will Ferrell clearly showing the importance of avoiding phone use at dinnertime. See what your kids think. Do they find it funny? Does it hit close to home? Are there changes you want to make in your family dinner technology rules after watching it?
- **Establish a regular plan:** A plan can lead to more meals together. They don't have to be perfect meals, perfect times, or perfect schedules. The point is to ensure the meals are eaten together.

Chapter 8

LEARNING

What we will cover

- Limitations of infant learning from screens
- How young children learn through screen media and how this contrasts with offline play
- Managing YouTube and navigating school-issued devices and educational technology
- Preventing dependence on AI

For years, educators have been excited about the role technology and media might play in children's learning. When it is designed well, media can provide educational opportunities, such as watching powerful documentaries, learning to code, or discovering new cultures in other countries. However, if media is designed around commercial goals, like advertising revenue, or is introduced too fast or carelessly, it can undermine learning while hiding behind educational claims. This chapter takes an ages-and-stages approach to helping you understand what children can (and can't) learn from media in infancy and early childhood. We also cover the school years and how to navigate school-issued devices, AI, and educational technology, which we will refer to as *ed tech*, to make sure that it is supporting, rather than distracting, from kids' growth in knowledge. We will focus on how adolescents learn directly from media in later chapters that focus on specific topics, including body image (see Chapter 12); violence, aggression, and hate speech (see Chapter 13); and risky behaviors (see Chapter 15).

Definition

Ed tech is shorthand for *educational technology*. It includes digital tools such as apps, virtual classrooms, educational software, learning management systems, and online platforms implemented by schools. It also includes software such as online courses and hardware such as laptops and tablets. It does not include the multitude of consumer-facing apps and videos that make "educational" claims that aren't delivered through schools.

Infancy and Toddlerhood (1-24 Months)

This is a period when parents feel exhausted and a bit overwhelmed adjusting to their new life caring for another human being. The cycles of feeding, sleeping, cleaning, diapering, and holding can make you forget who you were before having kids. Building infant developmental skills doesn't need to be flashy or even pretty. Sometimes the most ordinary things you do with your infant are extraordinary—sitting them on your lap and gurgling back and forth, bringing out belly laughs with peekaboo, putting toys in front of them during tummy time, or singing a lullaby you learned as a child.

Some parents share that they want to introduce screens to babies to educate them, so it's important to know the limitations of screens in this age range.

What Do Infant Brains Actually Absorb From Screens?

Infant brains are pretty amazing! They are made up of rapidly growing neurons and connections that help them coordinate their muscles, sit up, walk, clap, babble, pick things up, and explore the world with their hands and senses. However, one thing they can't do yet before age 18 months is decode symbols. Symbols are everywhere in digital media, and psychologists have found that infants struggle to understand that something they see on a screen (eg, a cat) represents something they might see in real life. They also have limited memory flexibility. Therefore, when they see a skill taught on a screen, they can't remember and apply that skill to their own life. Having a caregiver watch along to teach the skill can help with learning from screens in the toddler years.

The bottom line is that infants learn quickly and effectively from humans, not screens. When screens are on in the home, infants ultimately hear fewer words from their caregivers. This is why infants with heavier screen time practices have higher risk of language and developmental delays. Infants may seem like they are staring at the lights and sounds on a screen—because their attention is entrained very well by those stimuli—but they're not actually absorbing educational material.

Why Do Some Parents Allow Infants to Watch Screens?

Infants' first screens are usually TVs. In the grand scheme of things, a TV is a more appropriate device than a phone or tablet because it allows an adult to co-view or monitor the programming. Parents often share that their main motivation for infant media use is to allow for a break themselves, such as to get some "me time" or to catch up on chores. Research suggests that a brief TV break of high-quality programs, such as *Sesame Street* or PBS KIDS, is not linked with any developmental problems. So in the spirit of good enough parenting, there is no need to feel guilty or shameful about occasional brief TV usage with your infant. The key is being intentional so that it doesn't turn into a long, daily habit.

Should Babies and Toddlers Have Tablets?

This is an easy answer—tablets are not needed for infants. There's no developmental need for a tablet, and it will be too tempting to use it all the time to occupy a fussy baby. If a relative buys your baby a tablet, put it aside until after age 2 or later.

The Market for Baby TV Programming and Video Content

YouTube has made a market—and billions of dollars in ad revenue—off parent exhaustion. Over the past 10 years, there has been an explosion of kid-focused content, with primary colors, happy smiling animals, and big red text advertising how long your child will be occupied (60 minutes! 2 hours!). Content creators realized they could make a profit with cheaply made but mesmerizing kids' content, and the algorithm recommends content that is clicked on and watched the most, so there are now millions of hours of kids' content on YouTube. I (Jenny) have done a lot of research on what little kids are watching on YouTube and have not found much educational value in it (see Research Corner: Why Are Young Children Watching So Much YouTube? section later in this chapter). For infants especially, I would avoid it.

"I'm an exhausted parent who sometimes uses screens with my children, and I don't want to be judged. What do I do?"

Like we say many times in this book, there are many ways to do this right. The following are a few options:

- **100% screen free.** Don't have a TV in the room where you play with your baby (or at least keep it turned off), place your phone in another room, and only use video chat to connect with distant friends and family. Read only print books, keep all toys nonelectronic, and put on music to sing along with. Use your phone and watch your favorite shows when your baby is asleep. Pay attention to your stress levels, though—if you are feeling too much pressure to make everything "perfect" and organic, and are not actually enjoying parenting, rethink your approach.
- **Occasional snuggles while co-viewing.** With your infant, watch a music video or something you find beautiful and inspirational or something that calms you, and talk or sing along. It could be a soccer match or basketball game; a nature video; or a music video from Hepcat, a ska band I (Jenny) used to tour with (great dancing music!). We once were asked a great question at

the American Academy of Pediatrics Center of Excellence on Social Media and Youth Mental Health by the musician mom of an infant—she wanted to know whether it was OK to show her infant symphony videos. How cool! We recommended that she be intentional and make sure this wasn't the main way she engaged with her baby; no parent needs an algorithm to tell them how to sing and play with their children. Part of raising a young child is tapping into your own creative mind and remembering what it felt like to be a kid.

- **Regular, brief high-quality programming.** We've worked with a lot of parents who feel totally depleted in raising an infant. They feel that their day is dominated by meeting someone else's needs. It's common to struggle with depression or anxiety, isolation, or pain while trying to raise a little human in a society that doesn't provide a lot of early life support. Parents want to know whether it's OK to set their infant in front of a screen while they practice self-care or do the dishes. When you find yourself in this situation, don't panic. Evidence, including a meta-analysis of early childhood screen use research published in the journal *JAMA Pediatrics* in 2020, showed that watching brief high-quality programs is not linked with any developmental problems. It's especially helpful if parents talk to the baby about what is happening on the screen. The key points to keep in mind are (1) avoid going down a slippery slope of 30 minutes turning into several hours of baby media per day and (2) avoid starting with lower-quality YouTube videos that are engineered to grab attention.

Early Childhood (2–5 Years)

Early childhood contains many bursts of development, such as language, emotions, and movement like running and climbing. It is a period when children start to slowly seek independence from parents. It's typical (and good!) for them to want to explore, do things on their own, and then check back in with their trusted grown-up—this is called *secure base* behavior. This helps toddlers build a sense of security that they can handle things on their own, with the knowledge that you will be there for them when they need you. It's also a time when children are trying to master emotions on their own (see Chapter 10) but need your help in figuring out what they are feeling and how to manage it.

TV and Videos: What Is Considered Educational?

Although young children don't *need* screen media to learn or prepare for preschool, around 2 years of age their brains are finally able to absorb facts and knowledge from well-crafted TV programs. Studies evaluating the effect of PBS KIDS shows have shown that they can teach little kids: Viewing *Martha Speaks* led to more vocabulary words, watching *Daniel Tiger's Neighborhood* with caregivers led to better emotional skills, and watching *Between the Lions* helped kids learn early literacy skills such as identifying letters. If you're going to allow your child to spend time with media before age 5, these types of shows are your best bet.

Video platforms such as YouTube contain a lot of low-quality videos that might advertise themselves as educational in the title, but when you view them, you see they are what we refer to as *shallow educational content.* They may be glitzy or satisfying to watch (eg, a "kidfluencer" sorting toys and naming their colors), but they are mainly trying to grab attention to make advertising dollars.

Are Tablets Educational?

In early childhood, tablets are not needed for educational purposes. In fact, a study published in *JAMA Pediatrics* in 2024 found that 3- to 5-year-olds with more tablet use had more expressions of anger and frustration 1 year later than young children who rarely used tablets did. It's possible that young children with tablet access have worse sleep, are used to tablets managing their emotions (see Chapter 10), and/or gain access to inappropriate content. In my (Jenny) 2020 study, published in *Pediatrics*, we found that many young children accessed inappropriate apps on their tablets, such as games that let kids extract rotten teeth, pop cartoon pimples, crash cars, shoot guns, or beat up a doll.

Research Corner | **Why Are Young Children Watching So Much YouTube?**

My (Jenny) lab studies YouTube—specifically, the videos that toddlers and preschoolers enrolled in my studies watch. If a young child watches YouTube regularly (which over half of young children do), we ask parents to send us links to the last 10 videos that their child watched. In a 2020 report with Common Sense Media, we found the following:

- Advertising was pervasive, occurring in 95% of early childhood videos. This matters because young children can't differentiate ads from shows, so they can be manipulated more easily. Ads are also distracting.
- Almost half (45%) of the videos featured or promoted products for children to buy, such as toys or YouTuber merchandise. Marketing firms know that if they want to reach young kids, they should include their product in a YouTube video.
- Videos contained negative themes such as violence (30%), bullying or pranking (20%), and sexual content (6%). (No thanks!)
- When we looked at the educational quality of the videos watched, only 25% had any educational content, but it was often shallow, such as a YouTuber naming the colors of the balls in a ball pit. Only 5% had high-quality educational content, akin to *Sesame Street* or *Daniel Tiger's Neighborhood.*

Overall, YouTube is a place where it's easy to find extremely satisfying, branded, fast-paced, and shallow content. This type of content gets a lot of clicks and therefore is recommended by the algorithm. If your child uses YouTube, you should monitor what they are watching and know that you may need to work a little harder to find the real educational content.

Here are some of our YouTube pro tips.

1. **No short-form video.** In early childhood, children should only be engaging with long-form content where they need to pay attention and follow a storyline.
2. **No AI-generated content.** It's important for children to experience what human-created media feels like rather than becoming accustomed to the extremely satisfying and attention-grabbing design of AI-generated images and videos.
3. **Curated list.** You can make a playlist of the videos you want your child to watch.
4. **Avoid the junk.** You can block the YouTubers and channels you find annoying or shallow.
5. **Consider alternatives.** You could try an alternative video platform that doesn't rely on a recommendation feed or that has humans review all the videos before they are posted (eg, the Sensical app uses human review).

If you do allow your child to use a tablet, a good starting point is to set up parental controls so that your child can't download apps without your approval. These parental controls can also set time limits for apps and even downtime when the tablet can't be used. I (Jenny) usually share with parents to have the tablet "sleep" in another room away from the child's bedroom so that it's out of sight and out of mind for most of the day. Some children with autism or communication delays use an iPad at this age as a communication device, which can be very helpful. The advice we've heard from parents is to keep this "talkie" iPad as only a communication device—with no other games or apps installed to distract the child.

How Can Parents Find Truly Educational Media?

If you have a young child, there are a few things to look for that signal that an educational program or app can teach authentic skills.

- Can your child show the skill at another time or place? Researchers measure children's learning from media in terms of how well a child can transfer what they learned on a 2-dimensional screen

Research Corner | **Are "Educational Apps" *Really* Educational?**

Words such as *educational* and *early learning* have increasingly become marketing terms, making it difficult for parents to know what's worth their child's time and attention. To investigate this, my (Jenny) lab conducted a study published in the *Journal of Children and Media* in 2021 where we downloaded and played more than 100 of the most popular apps that called themselves "educational" through the Apple and Google stores. We evaluated them on 4 measures that child learning experts had created.

1. **Minds-on learning.** Does the app require the child to play a repetitive set of games, where their mind goes on autopilot while they engage in satisfying things like matching colors or tracing letters? Or does the app allow the child to come up with their own responses, follow their own imagination, and challenge themselves in new ways?
2. **Distraction.** Does the app have distracting features such as pop-up ads or buzzy bells and whistles or rewards that draw attention away from the learning goal (eg, a counting app that prompts you to tap all the creatures to make silly sounds)? Or do the interactive features help support the child toward the learning goal, such as providing hints about next steps in the activity?
3. **Meaningful experiences.** Is the app relevant to children's everyday lives, such as a potty-training app or showing ways to apply learning to the world around them? Or is it less relevant, such as a game where you count aliens or put makeup on pets?
4. **Social connection.** Does the app create a space for a parent or sibling to play along, for example, by allowing multi-touch inputs or turn taking? Or is it only trying to harness a single user's engagement?

When we reviewed all these features, we found that more than two-thirds of the apps contained low educational quality, even though they labeled themselves "educational." We concluded that many app developers want to make money off kids' time and attention, knowing that parents want their child to be occupied with something educational. Therefore, parents should have healthy skepticism when they see any app or video making educational claims.

to the 3-dimensional world around them. They need to be able to apply that knowledge even when not watching the show or playing the game—that is the true sign that the concept stuck. Think of a child who watches a math show such as *Odd Squad*, learns about fractions, and then uses that knowledge to talk about the amount of a pizza ($^3/_8$!) that they had for dinner that night.
- Another good sign of educational media is that it allows children to disengage and do non-screen activities. It doesn't try to get them to watch longer through clickbait titles or cliff-hanger endings. Educational media might prompt the child to go play or talk to someone around them. For example, Mister Rogers encouraged children to talk to their parents about what they learned. After *Curious George* episodes, there are prompts to go play with things they may have in their home.
- Educational media shouldn't feature a lot of ads, sponsored product placement, rude behavior, prompts to make purchases, or design tricks to make kids play longer.

Downside: How Technology Can Displace Reading and Play

If we had to pick the 2 most educational activities for young children, we would choose reading and play. This probably seems obvious to parents. But what we often hear from stressed and overworked parents is that a screen or device is the "easy button" that keeps households quiet and children occupied—that it takes more effort to carve out time to read or get outside to play. But here's why those activities are important—and practical ideas for making them happen.

Reading Builds Language Skills and Attention Span

Children and teens are reading for fun less than they did in the past. Data from the US National Center for Education Statistics in 2022 showed that only 19% of 9-year-olds read for fun almost every day, compared with 42% in 2020 and 53% in 2012. With 13-year-olds, reading for fun only happens regularly in 14%, down from 27% in 2012.

The fun and easy accessibility of digital media likely explains why fewer children are picking up books for leisure time, but it's also important to remember individual child differences. Reading comes easily to some children; if you have a bookworm who loves nothing more than to cuddle on the couch with a stack of new books from the library, count yourself fortunate. Other children find reading to be cognitively challenging—perhaps because they have a language delay or *dyslexia* (a reading-related learning disability)—or because they are still working to build up the attention span needed for getting through a chapter book. If a 5-year-old has the option of a high-pleasure, low-friction game on a tablet and an unfamiliar library book in front of them, it's not super surprising if they choose the tablet. The following are a few activities families can try to raise readers:

- Read and snuggle together. Every day if possible. Let your child pick out the books at times, and you pick them other times. Choose books that align with their mood, their experiences, or the season.
- Take weekly trips to the library to check out a variety of books and help your child find pleasure in a calm, quiet environment. Look for reading programs at your library. For example, many libraries have summer reading programs where a child tracks the books they read to receive prizes such as stickers and bookmarks. These programs are a great way to lean into reading.
- Listen to audio stories. These can start as audio-only stories on YouTube or a Toniebox audio player and work up to podcasts and audio versions of chapter books.
- Create a cozy space at home where they can easily plop down with a few different books, such as a beanbag chair next to their bookshelf.
- Ask your child's school for literacy instruction if your child is struggling to learn to read. This usually happens in a *response to*

intervention (RTI) format in which they receive higher levels of support based on whether they are improving from the prior level of support. Track their reading level in report cards or through communication with teachers and ask for a meeting if you see stagnation in reading scores.

- Role model reading print books, magazines, or newspapers. As written words online become more and more dominated by AI-generated text, help them recognize the importance of written publications that are created by human minds and creativity.

Play Builds Emotional Well-Being, Motivation, and Imagination

Play is essential to emotional well-being and learning but is often displaced by screen time. A lot of play can occur online, but here we point out a few ways that offline play shapes the way kids think, feel, and learn.

- The natural world has a different sensory profile, in terms of lights, textures, and sounds, than indoor spaces. This can have a regulating effect, particularly on children with sensory differences.
- When we spend time outdoors, our eyes focus on near and distant objects. Research shows that when kids spend more time looking at nearby screens, 18 to 24 inches away from their eyes, rather than spending time outdoors, they have a higher risk of *myopia* (nearsightedness).
- Time outdoors has a wilder aspect to it that can satisfy the risk-taking drive of children who love to make forts, climb trees, or explore (see Chapter 15 for more on risk-taking behaviors). If you want your child to appreciate nature and wildlife, make the outdoors a priority—anything from backyard time to playground time and biking to hiking in a local wooded area.
- Play lets your child's mind take the lead rather than following directions or being constrained by the design of a digital game. Digital play activities can be very open-ended (think of *Minecraft* or an illustration app) or very closed loop, where you can only do a restricted range of activities (eg, a puzzle game or *Space Invaders* type of design). In the latter case, a developer is always shaping your child's next move. In order to develop executive functions such as initiation, resisting distractions, planning, and problem-solving, it

helps to engage in activities where your child's mind comes up with the plan and executes it. This could be tabletop activities such as Play-Doh, arts and crafts, or LEGO. It could also be role-playing imaginative games like playing teacher, librarian, or dragon slayer or games where your children make up the rules.

We get it: Children may resist when they are asked to intrinsically motivate and make up games that fill their boredom. It's hard to create ideas from scratch. Think of it as developmentally helpful friction that a child may feel when asked to push past their boredom or to try a new activity. They may whine, but they can handle it. And over time, they will build the confidence that they can handle new challenges. (See Chapter 15 for tips to help motivate children who are resistant.)

Summing Up: Early Childhood

Like in infancy, there are several ways for young children to have healthy relationships with media.

- **100% screen-free.** Encourage screen-free time, but don't panic when watching occasional movies, sports games, or shows. Make sure they are age appropriate and something you watch together.
- **High-quality screen time.** Stick with educational content as much as possible: Embrace PBS KIDS and *Sesame Street* and other high-quality programs, with some Disney movies and other shows or movies in moderation. It's OK to have 1 to 2 hours of screens per day at this age, but we recommend that it be at a consistent time of day and to not allow an algorithm to pick what your child watches. If your child has a tablet, have only a few high-quality games on it (eg, LEGO, PBS KIDS, *Toca Boca*, and *Sesame Street* games scored high for educational quality in my [Jenny] research).
- **YouTube as part of the mix.** If your young child watches YouTube, monitor the content closely. Some parents make playlists that contain only the videos they want their child to watch. We have also heard from parents that they like introducing their child to videos they watched when they were little, such as *The Backyardigans*, *Bear in the Big Blue House*, *Mister Rogers' Neighborhood*, or *Little Bear*. This is great because these older shows are slower paced, and you will have fun watching along.

Intrinsic Motivation Versus Extrinsic Motivation

Video games have specific designs that motivate children to keep playing—new levels, rewards, in-game currency, or items like new skins or weapons. In a 2023 study from my (Jenny) lab, we found that these rewarding designs often pop up just at the perfect moment to keep users engaged in the game, such as at the end of a level or to encourage the player to come back every day. This is called *extrinsic motivation*—something outside of the child that encourages them to keep participating in an activity. If you've ever promised your child a tasty snack if they can stay well-behaved on a busy shopping trip, you've used extrinsic motivation. However, children also need to develop *intrinsic motivation*—the inner drive to start and follow through on tasks. Intrinsic motivation is crucial for getting through a school day, and it is shaped by positive experiences with inner rewards, such as the good feeling a child might get when coloring, laughing while playing a chasing game, or nailing the saxophone solo they have been practicing. Children with executive functioning deficits like attention-deficit/hyperactivity disorder (ADHD) and autism struggle with intrinsic motivation, which is why parents often use more behavioral rewards to help teach and reinforce positive skills with them. However, we don't want children to always need extrinsic motivation to accomplish tasks (eg, a child always asking, "What will you give me if I do that?"); we want them to feel a drive and a purpose that are inherently satisfying—which is what imaginative, creative, and physical play provide.

School Years: Elementary Through High School

We often field questions from parents worried about the amount of screen time their children experience in school. They wonder whether there is an ideal number of hours that screens should be used versus offline learning or if there is an ideal age when screens should (or shouldn't) be used in schools.

Some of this parental stress stems from the fact that ed tech tools and devices were thrust upon parents for remote learning during the COVID-19 pandemic. Schools scrambled to issue Chromebooks, help kids find Wi-Fi to log on to virtual learning, and move all their curricula onto online platforms. When many schools started reopening to full or hybrid models, families who were left in all-remote schooling struggled. My (Jenny) research found that Michigan elementary students who stayed fully remote through most of the 2020–2021 school year showed higher levels of sleep problems, had more emotional and behavioral problems, were less likely to have a best friend, and were more likely to refuse to do their schoolwork. Chromebooks and ed tech became a natural frustration point for hundreds of thousands of parents across the country.

Even years out from the start of the pandemic, a lot of ed tech has stuck around. But is it needed? And what is the best way to use it?

Neither Megan nor I is an educator, so we don't have expertise in teaching techniques or the different funding or curriculum challenges that schools have faced over the past 20 years as ed tech use has become more prevalent. But we have collectively treated thousands of patients with school-related struggles and this page to page 176 details how we see the benefits, problems, and potential solutions regarding ed tech.

Benefits of Ed Tech for Those With Learning Challenges

Children who are neurodivergent have been using ed tech for purpose-driven accommodations far before the pandemic. Children with dyslexia benefit from digital books that they can read, seeing the words highlighted, while listening to audio of the words read aloud. This needs to be paired with intensive reading instruction from a teacher, but it gives a child practice and allows for participation in reading books and related benefits in terms of imagination and learning. Children with learning disabilities benefit from daily practice of math or reading skills through evidence-based ed tech programs that provide a little gamification such as levels or characters, while also sending scores to the teacher to help them track the child's progress. Children with *dysgraphia*, a learning disability that affects handwriting and spelling, benefit from speech-to-text software that can transcribe their words, take notes, or help them structure and write essays.

In addition to these assistive technologies, many of our teenage patients have benefited from the platforms that organize their grades and assignments and communicate with teachers about late assignments. For some, this didn't exist before the pandemic, but it helped middle schoolers and high schoolers participate in more self-management and self-advocacy about their grades. At the same time, we've both had patients who stressed a lot when their teacher was late to update grades or respond to messages. Teachers are busy people! Our advice is to check these platforms no more than once a week.

It would be amazing if school districts or the Department of Education could publish the evidence underlying the most commonly used ed tech products so that parents could feel reassured that the screen time their child is getting during school hours is time well spent. However, this evidence can be found in a few different places, if you have the time and energy to go digging.

- The International Society for Technology in Education (https://iste.org/iste-seal) provides a seal to add to ed tech products that meet its standards. Here you can scroll through the different ed tech products and read their evaluation reports.
- The EdTech Index (https://edtechindex.org) is a database of thousands of ed tech products and what they intend to teach so that you can familiarize yourself with what your child uses; however, it doesn't provide evidence regarding learning effectiveness.
- Internet Safety Labs (https://internetsafetylabs.org) reports evaluations of apps and ed tech products, including what data these apps collect and who they share it with.

Downsides of Ed Tech

The negatives of tech use in school follow the same patterns that we see in terms of problems outside of school.

- **Displacement.** This could include students being on school devices during lunch periods rather than socializing, which can sometimes be driven by and enhance social anxiety; students completing assignments on their own devices, rather than participating in group-based collaborative work; and devices being used to occupy students during downtime or indoor recess, displacing time for social interaction or outdoor play.

- **Distraction or interruption.** Students might split their attention between their classwork and the multiple other tabs they have open on their computer. In the spring of 2021, I (Jenny) asked a school-issued device monitoring software company about the level of distraction it saw on students' Chromebooks during the pandemic. The answer: Teachers had closed over 50 million distracting browser tabs on their students' devices that year. Kids can feel really overwhelmed or bored in school—especially during remote learning—so it's not surprising that so many students followed the temptation to click on online distractions.
- **Inappropriate content.** Despite having filtering and safety software on school devices, kids find ways to access video game websites, AI platforms, or other inappropriate content. They often share tips on which websites are getting through filters, so school administrators play a game of whack-a-mole trying to shut down the distractions before another one pops up.
- **Difficulty transitioning.** Many of my (Jenny) patients with autism have struggled to transition from preferred activities on school devices to less-preferred learning activities. In some cases, we have had to ask for less device-based classwork, and more pen-and-paper assignments, to help the child stay behaviorally regulated during the day.

Studies interviewing parents of school-age children and teens suggest that school-issued devices can be a source of arguments. One parent shared sentiments that might feel familiar: *"[My child] didn't have a device until we had to get one for school, and now he's got this Chromebook that I've got to try to control.... I had no intention of him having a device at this stage. He has to do all his homework on it; then I've got to creep into his room and say 'Oh, that doesn't look like homework; it looks like another bloody YouTube video.' It's just another nightmare to manage."*

What Parents Can Do About Ed Tech

If ed tech feels like a nightmare in your home, you are not alone. Like with other forms of media, it's important to be involved, monitor, and advocate when it comes to your children's ed tech devices and activities.

- Have your child use their school-issued device in a common room in your home so that you can check in and make sure they are writing their essay, not watching a gamer video on YouTube.
- Find out which monitoring software is used for your school's devices (common ones are Securly and GoGuardian) and download the parent companion app. This allows you to track what your child is doing on their device. Explain to your child that you are doing this and that it may help them inhibit their impulse to pursue distractions.
- Talk openly about what distractions their classmates are engaging in. My (Jenny) younger son once told me that kids in his class chatted with inappropriate, sexy AI chatbots on a website that somehow got through the school device filters. I emailed the principal to ask her to look into whether the device filters could be tightened now that AI is another temptation on school devices.
- Ask if the device needs to come home at all for elementary-age students. Tell teachers and administrators your preference for pencil-and-paper assignments both at school and at home.
- Use your Wi-Fi controls to stop internet access to school devices during certain predictable hours (such as mealtimes) or before bed. For example, arrange it so that the device only has Wi-Fi between 4 pm and 6 pm, if that is the usual time your child does homework.
- Talk to your child's teacher or principal about providing students with non-tech alternative activities during indoor recess if you're worried about devices being used to keep kids occupied during downtime in school when they could otherwise be socializing. Inexpensive options include art supplies, decks of cards, or board games.
- Ask schools to tighten device filters, provide accommodations that minimize how much school devices are used during the day,

Research Corner | **Multitasking During Academic Time**

Whether students do their homework on paper or on a laptop, distractions are everywhere. As far back as 2007, studies have shown that students who use instant messaging while doing homework are more distracted. My (Megan) research team conducted a study in 2012 published in the journal *Computers in Human Behavior.* We sent text messages to college students 6 random times per day and asked what they were doing online. More than half of the time that students were using the internet, they reported that they were multitasking, meaning that they were using multiple media devices simultaneously. Distractions can now be all on the same device, whether multiple browser tabs open on a school-issued device or teens looking at social media or using their phones for news, texting, and listening to music while doing homework. Teens and adults with executive functioning challenges—such as difficulty with attention span, working memory, and impulse control—multitask more with media. Here's what parents can do, especially if you have a child with ADHD.

- Talk about media multitasking and how to resist it. Explain to your kids that it's totally normal to feel the urge to find something fun to watch when your brain feels overwhelmed with schoolwork, but it can make it harder to focus.
- Schedule breaks in homework time for kids who feel easily distracted. Set a timer and try 20 minutes of work, 10 minutes of break (movement, media, or a snack).
- Make a plan with their teacher to check in on their distraction levels or request that they do their work on paper instead if they are distracted on their school-issued computer or tablet during class. Another option is to track their off-task behaviors through the device's monitoring software and block the distracting websites (when possible).
- Role model "single-tasking." This means putting away your device at mealtimes, during family time, or while watching movies together.

and ensure that downtime is filled with reading or drawing—not gaming—when children with autism or ADHD struggle with distractions and transitions from devices in school.

- Talk with other parents about their concerns, discuss them at your Parent Teacher Organization, and advocate with the school district to improve their policies on school devices and ed tech.

Dos and don'ts of talking to teachers about ed tech

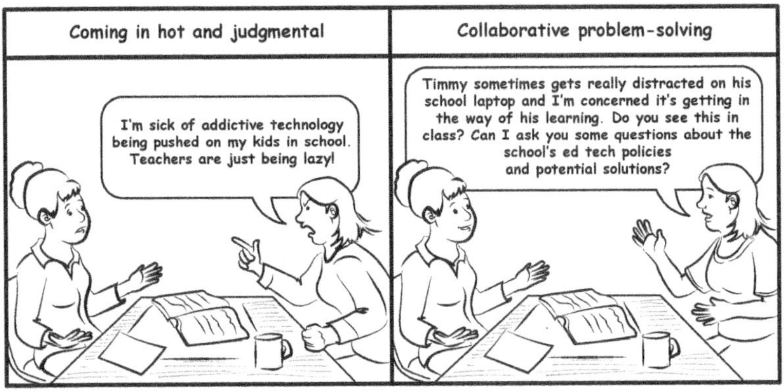
Coming in hot and judgmental
I'm sick of addictive technology being pushed on my kids in school. Teachers are just being lazy!
Collaborative problem-solving
Timmy sometimes gets really distracted on his school laptop and I'm concerned it's getting in the way of his learning. Do you see this in class? Can I ask you some questions about the school's ed tech policies and potential solutions?

Generative AI: What Effect Does It Have on Learning?

True learning in childhood and the teen years requires scaffolding, a concept we discussed in Chapter 1. Scaffolding involves supporting young learners in their *zone of proximal development* in which we provide challenges to help them accomplish and learn things they otherwise wouldn't have picked up on their own. Scaffolding is most effective when it happens within trusted student-teacher relationships; a great teacher knows what hints, motivation, or teaching approaches a student might need to help a new concept stick.

Our concern is that generative AI platforms (such as ChatGPT, Claude, or Gemini) are more easily used for spoon-feeding answers and off-loading cognitive work rather than for scaffolding. Yes, teens have found creative ways of asking AI chatbots to create tests for them based on their class notes. But many other teens use AI for essay writing, idea generation, or cutting corners in a way that could significantly reduce their cognitive investment in learning.

School Phone Policies: What Parents Should Know

More schools are rolling out personal device policies that restrict access or use of smartphones, smartwatches, or other devices that students may bring from home. These policies are important because smartphone use during school is associated with more distraction, poorer academic outcomes, bullying, and less engagement in learning. In my (Jenny) 2023 study tracking the smartphone use of 11- to 17-year-olds, we found that 97% of them used their phone during school hours. Phones were mostly used for entertainment, not for learning purposes. The most used apps were social media platforms, YouTube, and mobile games. Studies evaluating the effect of school phone policies that restrict use on school grounds in the United Kingdom (published in *Labour Economics* in 2016) and Spain (published in *Applied Economic Analysis* in 2022) have found higher test scores and lower rates of bullying.

In my (Megan) research surveying US parents in 2024 (when many school districts were newly implementing phone policies), I found that kids who got in trouble for violating their school phone policy were more likely to have a parent who was texting them multiple times per day, have a chronic illness that influenced how much they needed to access their device or communicate with parents, or have a less restrictive phone policy at their school. This study was published in the *Journal of Adolescent Health* in 2026. As takeaways, parents should consider the following:

- Be careful about how often you text your child during the school day. On most phones, you can schedule messages so they send and arrive at the end of the school day.
- Have a clear plan of how you will communicate with your child during the school day, such as by calling the main office or by texting at a time that is allowed by the school.
- Ask for accommodation if your child has a condition such as diabetes that requires access to a smartphone-based glucose monitor. You can ask for accommodation on your child's 504 plan

or Individualized Education Program (IEP) that allows them to use their smartphone for these purposes.

- Advocate for the school to offer non-screen ways for students to connect socially (such as card games during lunch) and for students to self-regulate when upset (which is a main reason why kids use their phones during school, Jenny's study suggested).
- When your child gets home from school, they may want to catch up on missed notifications or messaging friends. Allow some time for this that works with their afternoon schedule, but don't let it interfere with homework, mealtimes, or sleep. Normalize being away from phones for longer stretches of time.

Critical thinking is a practice that involves learning to analyze, synthesize, and evaluate information. This is a crucial skill developed and honed in middle school, high school, and college, but it may be weakened by use of generative AI. A 2025 study conducted by Microsoft and Carnegie Mellon University surveyed 319 adult knowledge workers and reviewed the ways these workers asked AI for help during daily tasks. They found that when workers were less confident in themselves, and more confident in AI, they used less critical thinking in AI-assisted tasks. Workers with more confidence in their own skills used more critical thinking, even when AI assisted them. A key takeaway from this study is that if we can help children and teens be more confident in their own thinking skills without AI assistance, we can help them be more resilient in the face of increasing AI use in workplaces later on.

Another 2025 study, this one from the MIT Media Lab, focused on the use of generative AI in academic tasks such as essay writing and shed some light on the effects of off-loading thinking to AI. Students were randomized to either write an essay on their own or have AI assist them. Those who relied on AI to help them write the essay didn't use as much of their brain (based on EEG activation of different brain areas), felt less ownership over their work, and remembered less of what they wrote. We have spoken to many college professors who can easily sense when AI wrote an assignment; they are concerned about how AI tools like ChatGPT are being used as shortcuts and therefore undermine the deep learning that should happen in college.

By the time this book is published, generative AI will continue to have evolved rapidly, and we can't possibly anticipate all the parenting tips you may need regarding this emerging technology. However, we can provide suggestions on how to raise a resilient learner who can think for themselves, which may prevent them from becoming dependent on AI. Chapter 3 also includes recommendations for preventing emotional dependency on AI.

- **Help them from an early age to love human-generated art, music, and writing.** This can start with children's picture books and then evolve into listening to jazz and classical music, enjoying comedians, or going to museums. Talk about the artists and humans behind the creations to help children and teens appreciate the power of human creativity. When AI creates words or art, it predicts the most likely response based on all the data it was trained on. In other words, it provides an average, expected response rather than using creativity as we humans do! By honoring human art forms and all their spontaneity and quirks, children and teens will hopefully be better critics of AI-generated content.
- **Teach them that knowledge is more than facts.** Humans need wisdom and meaning, not just data points. This means that children and teens need to listen to their grandparents, aunts, or uncles tell stories; use their imagination to create their own ideas; and pay attention to teachers who help them see the big-picture connections in life. Because AI is a prediction engine, it doesn't know the larger context of who you are and how you've lived your life. Your family does. Make it a habit to have your children ask their grandparents about what life was like when they were their age: "What was school like when you were 12?" "When did you start shaving? When do you think I should?" "How did you ask a person on a date when you were a teenager?"
- **Help them to trust their own ideas and the value of their hard work and to build confidence in their own critical thinking skills.** If they study hard for a test, or work a long time on a school project, make sure to follow up on how it went. Don't only ask about what grade they got. Ask them, "What surprised you

about that topic?" or "How did you come up with that idea? What did your teacher think?" Ask to read their essay or see something they created for their art class.

- **Let them know that AI can be wrong and even give harmful advice.** There have been many reported cases of AI chatbots providing made-up facts and references and, as we mention in Chapters 11 and 15, giving advice on unhealthy behaviors or even self-harm. The developers of AI chatbots didn't consider the unique ways that teens might use these products, so they may not have designed enough safeguards to prevent an AI chatbot from promoting inaccurate, harmful, or dangerous content.
- **Help your teen recognize when they are off-loading thinking.** In middle school and high school, teens develop what is called *metacognition*—the ability to think about one's own thoughts. This critical thinking skill matures as teens become more abstract, reflective thinkers who can synthesize different pieces of knowledge, see the big picture, and form their own opinions. This is also an age when most teens who are neurotypical can start to self-manage their attention and study skills (rather than depending on a teacher or parent to always remind them). In middle school, students learn to get from class to class, organize their assignments, and think for themselves. During this time, AI use should be only with oversight from teachers, if at all. In the high school years, make sure that students know the school's and teachers' AI use policies. Some teachers will avoid it altogether. Others might allow use of it for limited purposes (eg, research, brainstorming, checking grammar). Check in with your teen about whether they feel like AI is a helpful tool or it's becoming a crutch. Ask questions like "Do you ever ask AI for help with things that you know you could do on your own?" One news story reported that a teen got in the habit of asking ChatGPT what to say to other people in everyday conversations. Instead of trusting his own ideas when asked a challenging question, he would duck into a bathroom and ask the chatbot what to say. Tell this story to your teen and see whether it resonates and what they would do if they were that person.

Like a lot of the technologies we discuss in this book, AI can be designed around children's unique developmental needs, or it can be designed to maximize time online and data collection. Schools can do families a favor by only adopting the AI technologies that have been safety tested and designed with specific educational purposes rather than providing access to commercial AI platforms that could be sources of distraction, cognitive off-loading, dependence, or unsafe advice.

Connecting the Dots

Being proactive about managing your child's ed tech is an important, albeit frustrating, part of the puzzle. As a parent, don't underestimate your power in being your child's first and most effective teacher. Through reading, playing, open dialogue, and helping them connect the dots to be a critical thinker, you can help them tolerate the extra cognitive work that comes with learning while also building confidence in their thinking skills. This will help them be resilient as AI becomes more integrated into daily life.

- **Talk to your friends and neighbors** about the distractions their kids are seeing on their school devices. Make a list of these and bring them to the school administrators to look for a systemic solution. Each parent shouldn't have to play whack-a-mole on their own.
- **Talk to your child about** AI and learning. Start by asking about what other kids are doing: "Do you see any classmates being too dependent on AI for schoolwork?" Follow up by exploring their opinions: "What do you think the risks of that are? What could go wrong?" Or try to be philosophical: "What worries you most about AI?" Follow up to understand whether those feelings influence their interest in or resistance to using AI.

Chapter 9

HEALTH LITERACY

What we will cover

- Why health literacy is important for children and teens
- How media can support kids' understanding of their bodies and health
- Health misinformation and its effect on kids
- Navigating health information and search results from AI chatbots

We are both pediatricians, so we think all bodies are cool. Both of us nerd out about the amazing way hearts, lungs, brains, skin, organs, and all other parts of our bodies work! We are grateful to be able to help kids learn about why they get sick, how they heal, and what they can do to stay healthy. Kids, on the other hand, may find health topics a little boring, so it's great to have accurate media help relay these messages to children and teens rather than having to rely on a cringey lecture from a parent or another adult! However, media can also be inaccurate or full of health-related clickbait, so *health literacy* needs to be coupled with a good dose of *digital literacy* these days.

Why It's Important to Understand Your Body and Health

Personal health literacy is crucial, even in childhood. The more children know about how their bodies work, the less anxious they will feel about what causes aches and pains, nervous stomachs, or a cough and fever. Being sick can feel scary, and knowledge can help kids cope. People with higher health literacy can get more out of doctor visits, stay out of the emergency room more, and advocate for what they need from their health care provider or health system.

Definitions

Personal health literacy was defined by the US government's Healthy People 2030 initiative as "the degree to which individuals have the ability to find, understand, and use information and services to inform health-related decisions and actions for themselves and others." Interestingly, Healthy People 2030 also called out **organizational health literacy** as "the degree to which organizations equitably enable individuals" to find and use good health information. In this chapter, we talk about the search engines, social media platforms, AI chatbots, and other online spaces where youth go looking for answers to health questions.

How Can You Teach Health Literacy to Kids?

For school-age children, I (Jenny) often draw out what is going on inside bodies to explain what is happening with asthma, anxiety, or (eek) puberty. At home, we have a wall covered with chalkboard paint where I have mapped out brains, lungs, gastrointestinal tracts, or bones as I try to explain particular health conditions to my kids. Reading is also a great source of health knowledge—my kids loved the graphic novel *Human Body Theater*, but there is a range of different books about growing bodies. In my (Megan) family, a favorite toy was the Visible Man (there is also a Visible Woman!) that had a clear plastic body filled with rubbery organs. The only way for the plastic body to click together was to put all the organs in the right places.

For teens, the internet, YouTube, and social media are increasingly their go-to source of health knowledge. They often seek it out independently—

and this is good! We want them to gradually take more ownership for their health care, such as asking questions about why they take medicine and why they are having certain symptoms. This helps young people engage in their health care and feel more confident in talking to their doctor. When patients don't feel like a partner in their health care, particularly if they feel that their concerns have been dismissed by a doctor, they are more likely to avoid the health system or look for alternative remedies. By starting to talk with children about how our bodies work from an early age, we can raise young adults who are not afraid to get all their questions answered from a doctor (even a busy doctor whose hand is on the doorknob) or speak up when they feel like their concerns are not being heard.

How Media Helps Kids Build Health Literacy

Here are a few examples of how we've harnessed videos or movies to teach kids about health.

Early Childhood

- Watch TV shows about going to the doctor or dentist, which can help role model how children can cope with anxiety. The COVID-19 pandemic was an anxiety-provoking time for all of us, and I (Jenny) had the chance to advise on an episode about Daniel Tiger dealing with going to the doctor on PBS KIDS.
- Potty-training videos and apps help spell out the whole confusing process to kids, including how to read your body's signals that you need to pee or poop, what to do while on the potty, and how to flush the toilet and wash your hands. And Taro Gomi's book *Everyone Poops* is a classic!

Middle Childhood and Teen Years

- During COVID-19, videos helped kids understand how germs infect the body, mutate, and spread between people and highlighted the importance of washing hands.
- As a developmental pediatrician, I (Jenny) often recommend videos about puberty and sexual relationships for patients with

autism and other developmental differences so that kids can absorb information about these sometimes awkward topics through visuals and stories.
- Curiosity about bodies increases during puberty, but teens also develop more self-reflection and awareness of how their bodies are feeling. What does this new hair mean? How do I handle pimples? Why do I have these headaches all the time? Showing kids and teens a few trusted sources, such as the American Academy of Pediatrics (AAP) After Hours Health website and the Nemours KidsHealth website (https://kidshealth.org), can help them have a trusted go-to reference when questions pop into their head. I (Megan) have provided these types of resources to teens, who often want a way to seek out answers to what may feel like embarrassing questions from a source that is private and accurate.

Should Kids Research Their Symptoms Online?

We recommend parent supervision when children choose to research health symptoms online. How much supervision depends on the child's age. For early and middle childhood, if you want to look something up related to your child's health (eg, *How long is norovirus contagious? What is this rash?*), use it as a role-modeling moment. If your child is sitting by your side, talk about how you choose which websites to read or videos to watch, which sources you skip (eg, avoiding any sponsored links), and how you evaluate the accuracy of any AI answer provided by the search engine (this could include clicking on the source links and reading them rather than just reading the AI summary). Websites can often list all possible diagnoses, from the mild to the fatal, so teach your child not to overreact. The goal is to learn a little bit about symptoms online and then use this knowledge to take next steps.

- "OK, the Centers for Disease Control and Prevention website says that norovirus can live on surfaces for over 2 weeks. This means that we should do a good cleaning of the house before Grandma comes over."
- "It seems like this rash could be due to a couple of different viruses or skin reactions. Let's call the pediatrician's office to get more help."

Doing some health searching online together also lets you show your child how you analyze different health messages, such as the difference between information you get from a pediatric website versus health claims made by an influencer. Here's an example of how unsupervised health symptom searching by kids can go wrong. My (Jenny) younger son, when he was 11, diagnosed himself with "exploding head syndrome."

What?

He said that he kept hearing a loud whooshing sound in his ears when trying to fall asleep, so he used his school laptop to search "Why am I hearing loud noises at night?" His search results explained that exploding head syndrome could be the cause (we still don't know exactly what that diagnosis is), and my son thought the name sounded cool and a little scary, so it stuck! This led to a cycle of nighttime anxiety, worries about exploding heads, and needing more support to fall asleep. We eventually got it under control by doing brief meditation exercises at bedtime, but I sure wish that I had been there to help him evaluate the online health information.

For teens, whose media use becomes more independent, we wouldn't expect a parent to be by their side whenever they search on or read health information online. However, you can teach them to start with a few trusted sources, such as the AAP parent website HealthyChildren.org, local university or hospital websites, or national mental health organizations (eg, Mental Health America, National Alliance on Mental Illness). Let them know that you are there as a sounding board, and cross-check the health information they find, no matter how sensitive.

How Do Teens Find Health Information Online?

Teens don't just search for health information online; it finds them too. My (Megan) research team did a study in 2023 published in the *Journal of Adolescent Health*. In this study, we collaborated with the AAP to host focus groups with teens to ask them about how they experienced health information online. We learned that adolescents were exposed to health information online both actively—by seeking it out on search engines or social media—and passively—when stories, ads, or social media posts popped up in their feeds or online.

Many teens described a complex approach for seeking health information (Figure 9.1); they would do a quick search to find initial answers and then cross-reference this information across other sites and sources. This is a great approach to checking that health information and advice are consistent, but it cannot always tell you that they are accurate. For that, you need other checks (eg, *Who is the author? Is the source a legitimate institution or some random website or influencer? Did they provide scientific references to back up their claims?*).

Adolescents seek online health information after various types of exposure to health information online, offline, and through their own identity or health condition. There are a variety of motivators and barriers that adolescents encounter when deciding whether to seek health information online. Teens will also search for health information on social media, which some teens use more than traditional search engines. Many teens have pretty sophisticated searching systems. For reasons described in the next section, we need to equip teens with a lot of health literacy skills if social media is their main source of health information.

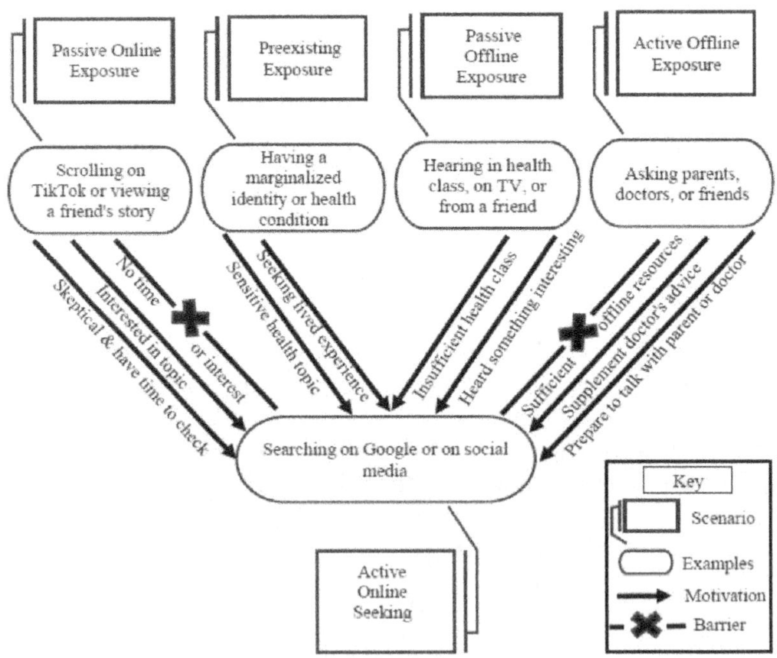

Figure 9.1 | **Motivations and Barriers to Online Health Information Seeking**

Source: Salerno A, Calvin A, Jenkins M, Moreno MA. Adolescent experiences with navigating health information on social media and beyond: using qualitative data to inform a model. *J Adolesc Health.* 2025;76(6):1018–1024. Used with permission.

Does this mean that online sources are replacing talking with parents or pediatricians? The answer is somewhat complicated. In some cases, a teen may look online for information before going to a parent or a pediatrician to get a sense of what may be happening. I (Megan) had a patient who said she thought she may have anxiety but wanted to get some background information before talking to her parents so she knew what the symptoms were and could be clear on what she was experiencing. In other cases, a teen may look online for information about a topic that is considered private or embarrassing in their family or community, which may be a topic such as puberty, sex, or mental health.

Health Misinformation

Health misinformation is more common than you might think. One 2021 systematic review published in the *Journal of Medical Internet Research* analyzed 69 other studies and found that health misinformation made up 43% of vaccine-related social media posts, pro–eating disorder suggestions were present on 36% of diet-related posts, and up to 40% of posts on chronic health conditions had misinformation. That means at least one-third of the time, you (and your teen) are going to have to have your "baloney detector" active while looking at social media posts about health. That's exhausting! Why is this so common?

What Drives Misinformation?

On any advertising-driven website or platform, the more clicks you get, the more ad dollars you can make. Therefore, websites and creators have an incentive to get people to click on their links and read their articles—and one effective way to do this is to say or promote outlandish things. You've seen links like this before.

- This one trick will change your life!
- 5 things your doctor won't tell you!
- 10 foods no nutritionist will eat!
- Lose belly fat while you sleep!

Some of them are too intriguing to ignore. The truth is that creators can *A/B test* different headlines (this means releasing 2 headlines at the same time, testing them against each other and seeing which ones generate more clicks) and then post the ones that grab the most attention. A key truth to teach your kids is that headlines are written to be attention grabbing and not to convey the whole complicated truth of the story. You'll need to read them through and think for yourself.

Health is a topic that garners a lot of misinformation online because it is a source of vulnerability and fear, and many Americans are frustrated with the health care system. People look to online sources for alternative answers about managing health and disease, and online content creators know that this translates into a huge market for clicks about vaccines, supplements, and promises of health optimization. A 2024 study from the University of Washington found that alternative health influencers make large amounts of money off advertising revenue, direct product sales, multilevel marketing, and brand deals, so they have a strong incentive to keep posting content that questions the safety or trustworthiness of medical care.

"The Chatbot Will See You Now"

It is mind-blowing how quickly AI chatbots such as ChatGPT, Copilot, and Gemini have been embraced by consumers since their introduction in late 2022. These products are powered by large language models (LLMs) that have been trained on information scraped from the internet and that have humanlike conversational styles that can synthesize and explain complicated concepts—health being one of those topics.

However, advocates (including the AAP) worry that this rapid uptake has not been balanced with sufficient safety testing: Was the model trained on any health misinformation? How biased is the output (eg, will it give different answers to a teenage boy versus a teenage girl)? If prompted, will it give inaccurate or dangerous health advice? If asked an esoteric question, will it *hallucinate* (fabricate) an answer? Will the authoritative, friendly, or supportive tone that some chatbots use make people more trusting, or even dependent, on AI for answers to all their unknowns?

Although it's possible to train a chatbot to provide safe and accurate health information, there have been several examples of people using general-use chatbots with potential negative consequences. One person asked AI what to do for a kidney stone, and AI told them to drink urine (ew…this is probably because the LLM was just predicting what word was likely to come next without understanding the larger context of the question). A 2025 study in the journal *Communications Medicine* found that when searchers used a fabricated prompt in a question to a chatbot (eg, asking for help with "Faulkenstein syndrome," which doesn't exist), the chatbot returned a whole bunch of fabricated misinformation in response. Therefore, if children or teens use a prompt that contains errors or odd questions, which they often do, they might get a very misleading answer.

Sycophancy in AI chatbots (which refers to when AI products are trained to agree with the user to build their trust and keep them engaged) can also be a serious problem. In a 2025 study, I (Jenny) and researchers from ParentsTogether Action and the Heat Initiative posed as teens using the chatbot platform Character.AI. When the teen (we) complained about their depression medication, the Rey chatbot (based on the popular *Star Wars* character) told the teen to stop taking their meds and how to hide it from their parents. As clinicians, we would much rather have an honest conversation with teens and parents about medication concerns than have a poorly trained chatbot meddle. As we will discuss in Chapter 10, sycophantic AI chatbots have also provided self-harm and suicide advice.

Practical Takeaway | **Using AI for Health-Related Searches**

When searching for health information with your child or teen online, you're likely to encounter an AI chatbot response. Specific websites (eg, the great special education resource website Understood.org) or apps (eg, the meditation app Insight Timer) may have their own custom-built chatbot embedded, so you should assume that your child is going to encounter these on their own personal or school-issued devices. Here are some key principles for using chatbots regarding health information without going down a risky rabbit hole.

- **Chatbots can be used for answers to basic questions, not final answers.** View chatbots as a starting point to understand things like headaches, sleep, acne, or other things your child or teen is struggling with. But like with other internet searches, there should always be follow-up conversations with parents or medical providers.
- **Chatbots can be used to help prepare for appointments, not replace appointments.** Chatbots can help you to generate a list of questions to ask the provider or to understand different causes of symptoms or different tests that are available. But you need the medical provider to put it all together with your individual history and physical exam and to follow up with you.
- **Understand that chatbots are prediction machines; don't assume that they are always accurate.** Chatbot output may seem "intelligent," but the computer science behind these products is simply word prediction. Always double-check other credible sources.
- **Don't upload medical records into chatbots.** Most chatbots have policies stating that they will use your prompts as training data, and you *do not* want your private medical data on a company's servers.

How to Support Teens' Digital Health Literacy (aka Baloney Detection)

Whether it is about health, science, influencers, or politics, there are several ways you can help your older child and teen be smarter about the information they see online.

- Teach them about classic clickbait tricks—bold claims, too-good-to-be-true promises, wild distorted photos, or slogans like "You won't believe this!"

- Help them understand the business model behind wellness influencers and the fact that their messages may be driven more by a profit motive than by accuracy.
- Help them learn to check in with their baloney detector about things they see online. This might show up as a feeling of excitement or even ick when reading something that doesn't seem legitimate.
- Show them a few trusted websites, and teach them how to check multiple health sources to see if they back each other up, just like what the teens described in my (Megan) previous study.
- Remind them that AI chatbots haven't been trained to provide reliable health information yet. AI information needs to be double-checked with a reliable source.
- Let them know you are there as a sounding board. If they read things online that they are not sure about, they can bounce their questions off you—and if you're not sure, ask your child's pediatrician.
- Remind them that AI chatbots use sycophancy, and be alert to ways in which they may foster relationship building with youth. (See Chapter 3 on parasocial relationships.)

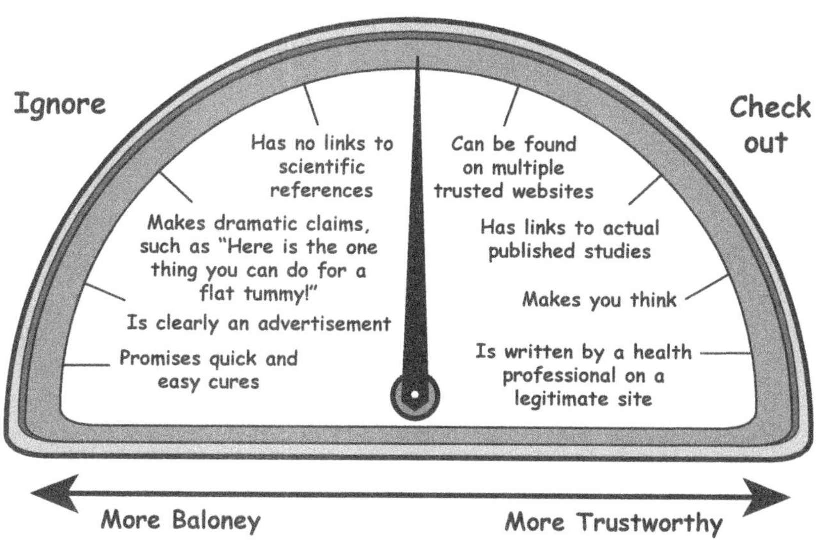

"Baloney Detector" for Health Misinformation

Connecting the Dots

We want our kids to be empowered to learn about their bodies and health through media, but we must prepare them to encounter a lot of online nonsense. Like with all topics in this book, the best thing you can do is talk about it and be there for them when they have questions. Health is a sensitive and vulnerable topic, so role model how to have honest conversations and build trusting relationships with doctors and health professionals. At the same time, help them have a healthy skepticism when consuming information that seems too good to be true.

- **Talk with your kids about** the wildest health claim or clickbait you've seen online. Who posted it? Why do you think they did? Who might believe it, and what are the consequences?
- **Talk with your friends about** the health trends you're seeing online. Are your friends seeing them too? Are you being profiled differently based on your online behaviors? Which health trends seem worth trying, and which seem like nonsense?

Part 3 | **Mental and Emotional Well-Being**

Chapter 10

EMOTIONAL WELL-BEING

What we will cover

- How media can support or undermine emotional well-being
- How the 5 Cs of Media Use affect mental health
- Practical strategies for keeping healthy emotional relationships with technology

The effect of digital media on youth mental health is probably the most hotly debated topic of the past decade. Various headlines can pull parents' attention in different, extreme directions. In this chapter, we focus on 5 factors that shape whether screens and technology have a net positive or negative influence on emotional well-being—the 5 Cs of Media Use that we developed with the American Academy of Pediatrics (AAP) Center of Excellence on Social Media and Youth Mental Health. These 5 Cs have practical takeaways that will leave you feeling like you have more insight into your kid's emotional processes and more ideas for keeping boundaries that protect emotional health.

Going Beyond Screen Time

When you look at children and teens averaged over a population level, and how their digital media use correlates with emotional or behavioral problems, the correlations are pretty small. As an example of the differences in effect compared with other health risks, a recent meta-analysis found that each hour of daily screen time correlated with an 11% higher risk of behavior problems in children 12 and younger; another meta-analysis found a 20% higher risk of depression in teens who used more than 2 hours of entertainment screen time per day. In comparison, smoking cigarettes is associated with a 1,500% to 3,000% increased risk of lung cancer—a pretty powerful link. The relatively smaller risk sizes in population-based studies of media use suggest that, across all kids, there are many other factors actively shaping youth mental health—poverty, adverse childhood experiences (eg, having a parent with a substance use disorder or who is incarcerated), the quality of their schools, or the strength of their relationship with their parents. Screen media use is only one factor, but it's a modifiable factor. This means that it's something families can work on to improve daily experiences, sleep, stress, and family time—so, it's worth the effort.

It's not that screen time doesn't matter, but it's only one dimension of media use that families need to pay attention to. At the AAP Center

Practical Takeaway | **Screen Time as a Marker of Higher Stress Levels**

We often think of higher screen time as having a negative effect on our emotional well-being. Sometimes, the reverse direction is true: We turn to our phones, gaming consoles, or TV more when we are feeling negative emotions and need an escape from daily stressors. Our AAP Center of Excellence on Social Media and Youth Mental Health Youth Advisory Panel members have taught us that parents could interpret higher screen time as a *marker* of a child or teen who is stressed out or struggling. If you notice that your teen's social media or gaming time has suddenly increased, maybe through family screen time settings or just noticing changes in behavior, make an effort to check in about stress. Our Youth Advisory Panel members recommend saying something like "Hey, I've noticed you are spending more time on Instagram this past week. What's up?" Ask open-minded questions about school, friends, and other life stresses; listen, reflect back what you're hearing, and discuss ways to solve the underlying problem rather than *only* limiting screen time.

of Excellence on Social Media and Youth Mental Health, we created the 5 Cs mnemonic as an easy-to-remember way for pediatricians and families to consider the aspects of media use important to well-being.

First C: Child

Media effects are not one-size-fits-all. You can probably think of a kid you know who is preoccupied with their gaming console or feels anxious without their phone and another kid who likes media well enough but easily separates from their phone when asked. There's emerging evidence that a child's *temperament* (eg, innate traits like how intense their emotional reactions are, how well they adapt to new situations, and their sensory sensitivities) and self-regulation abilities might shape their relationship with media.

In one of my (Jenny) studies published in 2014, we found that infants who were particularly fussy, demanding, and intense watched more TV than infants who were calmer and settled down more quickly. We guessed that this may be because parenting a fussy infant is exhausting and overwhelming, and looking at a screen can often quiet down fussing infants. To investigate this further, we published a study in 2016 in which we surveyed parents of toddlers about their motivations for screen use. As we had hypothesized, parents of fussier toddlers also reported higher rates of using screens to keep their toddlers calm and quiet.

Parents may wonder what the problem is with using screens as a calming tool. If it works, why not keep doing it?

To answer this question, we conducted a follow-up study in 2023 with 3- to 5-year-olds who we followed up for 6 months to understand the longer-term consequences of using media for calming. (The study was later mocked on *Saturday Night Live*'s "Weekend Update," which was the highlight of my [Jenny] career!) We found that when parents use screens more to calm their children, young children have more intense emotional reactivity over time. This was particularly the case for boys and children with more *surgent temperaments* (meaning that they have more intense emotions and impulsive behavior), who may need more support learning to handle big feelings.

What is the takeaway for parents? Being distracted by a screen in the midst of an emotional moment doesn't actually teach kids how to identify and manage that emotion. It may work well in the immediate moment (which is why it's helpful on planes or during other episodic, stressful moments), but off-loading emotion regulation to technology isn't a good investment in longer-term emotional health.

In teens, the same principles apply. I (Megan) conducted a 2022 study in which we looked for clusters of teens who seemed to be thriving on social media and those who were experiencing more problematic or risky use. The study found that struggling teens were more likely to have preexisting mental health conditions or less supportive relationships with their parents. This suggests that social media (or gaming or AI) might become an outlet that teens who are dysregulated seek out to help calm their emotions, escape from negative feelings, or withdraw from stressful family interactions.

Kids who are neurodivergent might also be more drawn to media because it contains endless access to their restricted interests. I (Jenny) have worked with many children with autism who love watching train videos, looking up facts like the capital of every country in the world, or speedily running *Subway Surfers* levels. For many kids with autism, interacting with the predictable patterns of screens or AI also feels easier than interacting with unpredictable humans.

For these reasons, parents of children who are neurodivergent or more emotionally sensitive or who have bigger emotional reactions may need to be particularly involved in supporting healthy tech boundaries and finding offline alternatives (see Fourth C: Crowing Out section later in this chapter).

Second C: Content

If you are a parent who uses social media, close your eyes and picture first a social media post that made you feel warm and happy (maybe a post about an adorable golden retriever or kitten), or a post that made you laugh out loud, and then picture something you saw in your feed that made you angry, disgusted, or anxious, maybe as part of doomscrolling. If you're not a social media user, think about a sitcom, news report, documentary, or reality show that stirred your emotions. Got those mental images? Great. These are perfect examples of how the content we consume—meaning, the images, stories, and messages in media—can deeply affect our emotions. This can occur over short time frames or longer time frames if you keep seeing the same types of content over and over.

Helpful Content

Media content can lighten people's moods in the moment or have long-term positive effects through teaching about emotional well-being. A 2025 randomized study asked 1,001 adults to watch different social media content for 5 days: They were randomly assigned to 1 of 2 groups. One group consumed professionally produced inspiring content, comedic content, or guided meditation. The other group was asked to scroll self-selected mobile media content. Those who watched the inspiring content (eg, an underdog story about a cancer survivor who climbed Mount Everest) or did the guided meditation had higher hope and lower stress. Interestingly, comedic content didn't change stress levels over time. Another 2025 study surveyed almost 7,000 adults who watched online cat videos and reported that cat-related content gave them more energy and positive feelings. If you've ever laughed with friends or family over these types of videos online, you know why people keep turning to social media or online videos for a mood boost.

Thoughtfully crafted videos, movies, and games can also teach emotional skills. One 2017 study of young children with autism spectrum disorder found that when they watched *Daniel Tiger's Neighborhood* with their parents and used skills like "when you feel so mad that you want to roar, take a deep breath and count to 4! 1…2…3…4," they had significantly better emotion regulation over time. In clinic, I (Jenny) regularly tell families to watch shows that teach about emotions, which is a complicated topic. I particularly like the Elmo *Belly Breathe* video, which teaches children how to breathe to calm down big emotions, as well as the movies *Inside Out* and *Inside Out 2* to build insight into emotions, kids' minds, and relationships.

Funny, supportive, or inspirational content or messages made by friends (see Chapter 2) also support emotional well-being and are a big reason why teens are drawn to social media.

High-Pleasure, Low-Friction Content

Are satisfying slime videos and unboxing videos OK? Are weird AI-generated *slop* videos or *brain rot* types of videos harmful if all they contain is fluff or entertainment? It's important to talk about this type of content, which sometimes can be a benign way to pass time and escape, but at worst these videos sometimes have hidden dog whistles or nihilistic messages that nothing matters. *Content farms* are social media or video channels that churn out a lot of low-quality, attention-grabbing content by reposting popular videos with catchy modifications, such as "Top 5" lists or split screen posts with videos layered next to each other (if you don't know what this means, consider yourself lucky—these videos are pretty overstimulating). Content creators who make these types of videos know that teens spend a lot of time online, have a harder time resisting attention-grabbing design, and can be a reliable source of ad revenue. A 2026 *New York Times* article highlighted how creators are even targeting young children with meaningless AI-generated cartoons featuring nursery rhymes, knowing that toddlers sometimes watch hours of these videos, which will bring in advertising dollars. We think that manipulating viewers' attention for profit is unethical, and your teen might feel that way too.

Call it by a name, like *brain rot* or *slop*, so that your kids and teens will be better at identifying it and how it makes them feel and deciding how much to block it in their feed or on YouTube. Talk about the business model behind it, which is unfairly trying to capture a child's or teen's attention for money. From a practical standpoint, let your teens know that the more they engage with this content, the more it will show up in their feed—and therefore crowd out other, helpful content that might have a more positive influence on their emotions.

Harmful Content

As we discuss in other chapters, harmful content and contacts are a main mechanism by which media has negative effects on children and teens; these include harassment from peers (see Chapter 2), body image content (see Chapter 12), violence and hateful content (see Chapter 13), risky content (see Chapter 15), and sexual exploitation (see Chapter 15). Numerous families have taken legal action against social media companies after their child experienced harm or died by suicide after consuming negative content online. When reviewing their child's or teen's social media history, bereaved families found pro-suicide content encouraging and instructing self-harm, content showing teens how to hide their eating disorder behaviors from their families, or anonymous harassment messages.

Although some social media companies have indicated that they now filter such content from teens' accounts, multiple investigations suggest the filters aren't fully effective.

Teens say that even content that doesn't violate social media content policies—like a feed concentrated with idealized beauty images—can make them feel negative about themselves. Algorithmic recommendations in feeds can amplify a developmentally typical interest (eg, beauty) into recommendations of posts that induce negative social comparison and make teens feel "less than." This is why many teens say they work hard to curate their feeds—for example, blocking, muting, or down ranking content that upsets them—or take breaks during times of intense world events (such as wars or shootings) that may flood social media.

Tech Corner | **Designing Feeds for Better Emotional Well-Being**

Algorithmic feeds are presentations of recommended content that are determined by a computer's automated decision-making. This decision-making, or how the algorithm is trained or tuned, is determined by the platform. Most critics of social media worry that algorithms that are trained on engagement—meaning that their goal is to recommend content that will attract the user's attention and keep them on longer—have been the source of multiple problems, such as extreme content (as well as misinformation and political polarization) being recommended to kids and teens. How could feeds in social media and video games be better?

- The feed could be turned off entirely. Sometimes teens may just want to chat with friends and not need to resist the distraction of a feed during times like school or bedtime.
- Feeds could be unavailable—or more difficult to access—during certain times of day like school hours.
- Different feed versions could be available, like TikTok's STEM feed, which is a feed focused on science, technology, engineering, and

mathematics content. Teens who follow this feed have it appear as a tab at the top of the app so they can jump right into this content that some of my (Megan) patients have called "informative" and "inspiring." In Europe, teens have the option of flipping to a "friends" feed, where only content from their friends shows up.

- Feeds could be trained to elevate content that the user says provides meaningful value to them rather than elevating whatever grabs their attention.
- Users could be given controls or settings to easily filter out AI-generated content.
- Advertisers could request to only show up on meaningful high-value feeds or only during certain times of day for teens. This would reduce the monetary drive for platforms to show ads to teens next to misinformation content or during disruptive times of day (eg, school hours or overnight).
- Our AAP Center of Excellence on Social Media and Youth Mental Health Youth Advisory Panel recommends that social media and gaming platforms, as well as smartphones, have timers that let teens set an intention for how long they want to use the product. When the timer goes off, it should be coupled with reminders for what else the teen indicated they would rather be doing, such as sleeping or going outdoors.

Third C: Calm

As we mentioned, frequently using media to escape or distract from negative emotions or social experiences can weaken kids' (and parents') skills of tolerating distress, building insight into what they feel and why they feel that way, and learning how to handle that feeling. Managing emotions is not easy—it takes practice!

For this reason, we recommend that kids and teens have what we call a *calming toolbox*—a go-to list of activities that helps them unwind a tightly coiled nervous system. For younger kids, I (Jenny) recommend using a color-coded visual like The Zones of Regulation, which helps kids identify how their brain and body are feeling in terms of colors: blue = bored, sad, or tired; green = calm, focused, or content; yellow = anxious, agitated, or excited; and red = angry, frightened, threatened, or out of control. At first, parents or therapists may need to help children name their color zone and pick from a list of calming choices (such as getting a hug or listening to music), but eventually kids can start to do this for themselves.

In the tween and teen years, micromanaging their emotions in the heat of the moment is not going to be helpful or effective! Talk to your teen when things are calm so that you can decide on a few activities that help them calm down. Parents and kids tell us that the following ideas are their most effective go-to activities:

- Listening to music or a meditation audio. This could be on a phone, but you could also invest in a record player, a CD player, or an MP3 player that they can use to listen to music that aligns with their mood or cheers them up.
- Spending time with a pet. This can be sensory and relational and provide unconditional love.

Research Corner | **Using Tech to Improve Mood**

In a 2024 study published in *Cyberpsychology, Behavior, and Social Networking*, my colleague Dr Matt Minich and I (Megan) texted adolescents at multiple intervals during the day to ask whether they were using their smartphone, what they were doing, and their mood rating before and during smartphone use. Adolescents reported mood improvements during smartphone activities, particularly when they were listening to music, podcasts, or audiobooks. This study suggested that teens may reach for their phone to help when their mood is low. Parents can help teens reflect on which smartphone activities usually help improve their mood in the moment versus which ones add to their stress.

- Moving their body. Walking around the block, dancing, doing yoga, going for a run, and doing sensory exercises such as wall push-ups all help the body send calming signals to the brain.
- Spending time in nature. Being outside provides new sensory input and can help kids get out of their heads and refocus on their natural surroundings.
- Talking it out. After calming down, let them know you're there for them and can help unpack how they were feeling.

Fourth C: Crowding Out

Too much media use starts to displace the things that keep us sane, emotionally connected to each other, or engaged in our community. We cover these in other chapters—family connection (see Chapter 1), peer relationships (see Chapter 2), sleep (see Chapter 5), and physical activity (see Chapter 6). This also has relevance for what families might want to "crowd back in" when they set new boundaries on media use. In my (Jenny) practice, I have discussed the following strategies with families:

- Instead of everyone being on their phone in the car, keep phones at home or stash them away and use the ride as a time to talk about school or life updates. For a long drive, consider an audiobook to listen to together.
- If video games are stretching on too long and interfering with completing homework, set a time limit that reduces video game usage and fill that time with your child having a dedicated space to do homework, maybe coupled with a snack and a nearby parent or sibling to help if they get stuck.
- Instead of allowing teens to be on their phones in their rooms for the entire weekend, arrange some activities such as bowling, a movie, taking the dog for a hike, or cooking together.
- If reading for fun isn't a regular habit for your family, "crowd it in" by having books and graphic novels around the house from a weekly library trip, order a monthly subscription to a magazine, or have a paper newspaper delivered daily or on Sundays.

- Making art is good for mental health, and it's worth the effort to set up an art cubby or space with whatever you or your child likes to create with—pencils, markers, paint, clay, or sewing or knitting supplies.

How tech can crowd out life

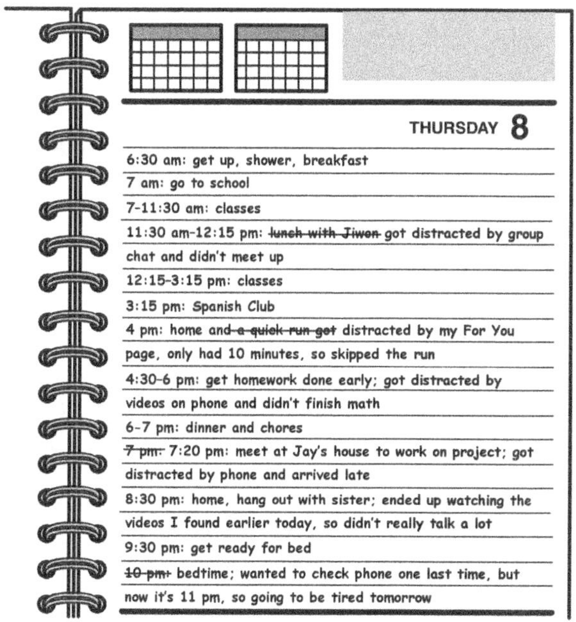

Fifth C: Communication

How we communicate about technology influences how our children think about it. Is it a forbidden fruit? Is it something you can turn on whenever bored and never need to think critically about? Is it something that causes arguments, or do you avoid talking about it altogether?

We recommend communicating with kids about media early and often. Technology is an embedded part of our environment and, as we've said before, isn't always created with the needs of families in mind. By seeing ourselves as media mentors and coaches, rather than as the media police, we can help our kids build digital literacy and be savvy about everything from ads to online predators to *flexing* (boastful or aggressive) influencers.

These conversations shouldn't be lectures. You can certainly speak your mind and discuss your own highs and lows with technology but also leave space for your child to share their thoughts. Curiosity is your best friend in these conversations—you may learn a lot about how your child is coping with friends, their passions, or their worries about the world or where their vulnerabilities lie. For teens who are reluctant to talk at first, use indirect approaches such as talking about what their peers are doing ("Who in your class is online too much?") or tech-related news ("Did you hear about that tech CEO scandal?").

Throughout this book, we talk about the importance of boundaries, using parental control settings, and being consistent about technology having a time and a place, but it's important that these boundaries be coupled with warmth. In parenting research,

- *Authoritative* parenting (high limits and high warmth) is most highly linked with child emotional well-being.
- *Authoritarian* parenting (high limits without warmth or explanations; my-way-or-the-highway mentality) can lead to more teen anxiety and defiance.
- Conversely, an overly *permissive* parenting style (high warmth, low limits) can open children and teens up to too many online risks, as does a *neglectful* parenting style (low warmth, low limits).

It's OK to feel worried about your child and the digital world, but if you come into these conversations too "hot," your child may withdraw. Choose times to communicate about technology that are low-key, such as when driving together, when watching movies or shows, or when you have other downtime.

What If Your Child Crosses a Line?

All kids will at some point make a mistake, cross a line, or break a rule when it comes to technology use. Consequences are needed when your child crosses a line, but the more you make these instances *natural consequences*, rather than harsh punishments, you can turn them into learning moments for your child. Remember that the word *discipline* comes from the word *disciple*—it's more about *teaching* than shame.

What are natural consequences when it comes to technology? The following are some examples from my (Jenny) parenting treasure trove:

- My older son, during the height of the pandemic, snuck a tablet I had brought home from my research lab and watched a bunch of the popular *MrBeast* YouTube videos on it overnight in his bedroom. *MrBeast* videos use a lot of attention-grabbing hooks (Lots of money! Trending challenges! High stakes, drama, and intrigue!) to engage viewers, and these tactics are especially effective on kids. I had a hunch that my son was not sleeping well, and when I was cleaning his bedroom, I found the tablet hidden in an empty shoebox!
    - **Learning moment:** We talked about why *MrBeast* videos are such clickbait and are difficult for a 10-year-old to resist and why dishonesty and sneaking something that's not yours is not OK. My family still calls this the "*MrBeast* Moment" when we want to jokingly refer to a time where we lost control over engagement-optimized media.
    - **Consequence:** All online activities had to be done in a common room (our living room), including use of his Chromebook for online school, rather than in his bedroom. We generally find that it's more social and easier to monitor what the kids are watching when it's on a screen in a common space.
    - **Tech limit:** I removed access to the tablet by returning it to my lab.
- My younger son has perfected the skill of finding distractions on his school-issued Chromebook, and it drives me up the wall. When he was in seventh grade, I got a call from his science teacher letting me know that he was distracted during class. I checked the school device monitoring software app on my phone, and it showed that he was playing a knockoff *Minecraft* game. (Note: I don't routinely check this app, as it's a lot of work to keep track of distractions. I wish the software would just filter out. More on this in Chapter 8.)
    - **Learning moment:** We talked about why he was playing video games in school, and he stated that some of the teachers allow it (this science teacher didn't, he learned), which was news to

me. We talked about the fact that knockoff video game websites can be full of viruses or predators, and it's really important that he use his Chromebook for assigned work only.

- **Consequence:** We told him that if we saw that he was playing video games while at school (which we could monitor through the monitoring software app), he wouldn't be able to play video games at home, which is his favorite weekend pastime. It worked!
- **Tech limit:** We went through his device monitoring app and blocked all of the gaming websites he had visited. We realize this is a game of whack-a-mole, and as we covered in Chapter 8, schools could really help families by providing more tech limits on school-issued devices.

Media Strategies and Planning

"I'm Raising a Sensitive/Dysregulated Young Child. How Does This Affect My Media Planning?"

If you are raising a more emotional, sensitive child, rest assured that they can grow up to have big hearts and be passionate advocates with creative minds. But you also need to make time and space for them to practice pausing, identifying emotions, and learning coping strategies rather than showing their emotions through blowups or shutdowns. It will be tempting to manage a lot of their behavior through the comfort of screens, but this can get in the way of learning how to tolerate distress.

The following are some practical strategies to consider in early childhood, when it is easier to start off with more limits to prevent problems rather than trying to peel back media use after it's become a problem:

- Avoid media with high-pleasure, low-friction content, which may quell behavior but also create habits that are hard to break. This may mean having minimal tablet time (as we review in Chapter 8, app stores are full of high-pleasure, low-friction apps) and little to no YouTube. Stick with long-form content from PBS KIDS, *Sesame Street,* Disney, Noggin, and other creators with backgrounds in child development.

- Keep media at predictable times of day or days of the week rather than providing it whenever your child asks.
- If you feel at a loss for effective strategies to manage behavior, see a therapist who can work on relationship-supporting, self-regulation, and behavior modification approaches.
- When your child eventually gets their first phone, start with fewer functionalities (like talk and text only), and then allow more apps as they show more emotional growth.
- As kids become older, consider mindfulness or calming apps as part of their media use.

"My Child Was Diagnosed With a Mood Disorder/ Disruptive Behavior. How Does This Affect My Media Planning?"

Kids and teens with mental health conditions are at higher risk of having problematic relationships with media, as we discuss in more detail in Chapter 14. The following are some things you can try to not fully restrict your child from media but also be able to monitor and build their insight into how media affects them:

- Consider emotional reactions. Kids with depression or anxiety might have more intense emotional reactions to what they see online, whether it be the news or social media. Help your teen understand how they react emotionally to media. Should they try to avoid horror movies to preserve their sleep? Should they take a break from social media if it's making them feel worse about themselves?
- Help them understand that their interests are often targeted on social media. For example, teens who seek out more beauty or fitness content might come across content that makes them feel worse about their body image. Teens who seek out more violent or morbid themes might come across more depressive content. If this happens, encourage your child to curate their feed or perhaps take a break from certain platforms.
- Try to keep video games more based on strategy or competition rather than violence.
- Make sure their devices can't access risky activities like the dark web or AI chatbots.

Tech Corner | **AI Chatbots and Mental Health Advice**

Almost three-quarters of teens are using AI chatbots, ranging from ChatGPT to role-playing AI companions like on Character.AI. A 2025 study published in *JAMA Network Open* surveyed more than 1,000 12- to 21-year-olds in the United States and found that 13% reported using AI chatbots for mental health advice. Almost all of these teens found the AI advice somewhat or very helpful.

Data directly from teens' devices paint a similar picture. A 2025 report from Aura, an internet safety company that monitors family devices, used data from more than 3,000 kids' devices and found that many teens use AI chatbots regularly. Of these, 42% used them for emotional support.

Research from the Harvard Center for Digital Thriving suggests that teens seek out support from AI because it is nonjudgmental and "listens" better than humans sometimes do. That's important feedback to parents—we need to be good listeners!

However, the risks of using AI chatbots for emotional support or mental health advice include the following:

- The chats are not private; sensitive information revealed when talking about mental health is stored on companies' servers and could be used to train their AI models or for marketing purposes.
- Popular AI chatbots do not have the mental health training or safety standards that human therapists or pediatricians do, including knowing when a young person is in crisis and needs emergency help. Therefore, they could fail to help a user when they need it most.
- Always talking to AI means that other loved ones don't know what the child or teen is going through or what is on their mind. This leaves family and friends unaware and makes it harder for them to know how best to help them.

- Chatbots have given harmful or even illegal advice, such as advice on self-harm or suicide.
- Users can become dependent on AI for answering their every question rather than learning to tolerate uncertainty or find other coping resources.

There will hopefully be free, safety-tested mental health chatbots available in the future, ideally with a human in the loop who can ensure that a patient is receiving sound advice. Until that time, we agree with groups such as the American Psychological Association that recommend using caution when asking AI to provide direct emotional support.

Connecting the Dots

The relationship between media and emotional health is complicated. Some types of long-form media offer more storytelling that helps kids and teens make sense of their experiences. Other types of media, especially those optimized for engagement, put kids at higher risk of coming across negative content, staying on too long, or causing conflict when they can't take their attention off the screen. There is a lot you can do to support emotional well-being in your kids.

- **Engage in an experiment:** Pick an activity that you and your children want to crowd back in to support your emotional well-being. It could be anything—a daily walk, more board games, having your kids help you prepare dinner, or some other activity that helps you feel connected. Pick a time of day when it will happen, and pick what type of tech use (especially the kind that adds to stress) that you each want to reduce. Try this for a week, or up to 3 weeks, and talk about how your mood is feeling with this new change. Did the experiment work? If not, what got in your way, and what else do you want to try?

- **Talk to your kids about** content that stresses you out. Is it bad news about the world? Influencer content that makes you feel less than? Ads that you think are inappropriate? By letting your children in your head a little bit, you can both teach them digital literacy and build emotional connection with you. Ask for their advice on how you can reduce exposure to stressful content—they might have effective ideas.

Chapter 11

SENSE OF SELF

What we will cover

- How a sense of self develops from childhood into the adult years
- How media can support, shape, or undermine a strong sense of self
- The balance of privacy and parent monitoring in teens' evolving sense of self
- What parents can do to help kids understand themselves and their unique strengths and challenges and how this shows up online and offline

What is sense of self? We devote a whole chapter to this concept because it is so important to human development, our relationships, and our interactions in the digital world. It's more than just self-esteem or identity. It's an inner experience of who you are; what matters to you; and what you bring to relationships with family, friends, school, and jobs.

In a digital world that is often trying to get your attention, some scholars have said "You are what you pay attention to." The goal of this chapter is to help your child or teen develop a solid sense of who they are and what they value so that they can stay strong while they face the headwinds and tailwinds of online spaces.

How a Sense of Self Develops

Early Years

In early childhood, the very first idea of *self* comes from our caregivers. Infant parenting experts describe caregivers as *mirrors*, helping a developing mind slowly come to understand itself. When parents mirror emotions back to their babies, talk about what they are doing, or label their feelings or experiences, young children start to develop *mental models* of who they are. So, if a child mostly is mirrored caring and responsive interactions, they come to understand that they are worth caring for. If a child is mostly mirrored feelings of anger or disgust from caregivers, they may internalize those thoughts about themselves. If a caregiver's attention is focused on technology, the infant may get no mirrored emotions at all. In fact, studies recorded parent and infant pairs while they played to see how infants responded when their playtime was interrupted by parents' attention being absorbed by a phone. On the videos, it was clear that infants found this digital disruption disorganizing—they fussed, wriggled their bodies, and tried to get their mirror back! This is likely one reason that young children of parents who use technology heavily have more behavioral difficulties.

Another approach that encourages a strong sense of self in early childhood is being *mind-minded.* We touched on this in Chapter 1, but let's revisit it because when *you* understand what's going on in your child's mind, *they* will understand their internal thoughts and feelings better. What are they struggling with? What are they excited about? If you see a challenging behavior, try to understand what is going on in their mind (ie, "looking under the hood") rather than immediately reacting. Be curious, say out loud what your hunch is, and help them find a solution: "Hmm, I think you're overwhelmed at this birthday party. It's busy here. Let's take a break together." This type of dynamic thinking takes a lot of brainpower, and research shows that when parents' minds are focused on technology—the latest news alert, funny social media video, or work email—there is less space for thinking about parenting.

Research Corner | **Parent Phone Use at Mealtimes**

In a study in 2018, published in the *Journal of Developmental & Behavioral Pediatrics*, my lab and I (Jenny) used recordings that families took of typical family meals to examine how parents used their phones during mealtimes. About one-quarter of parents used phones during meals, which matters because mealtimes are a common time when parents and kids connect about their day. All parents were interviewed with a method called the *Working Model of the Child Interview*, which asked parents to describe their child in 3 words, give examples of why they chose those words, and talk about how their parenting behavior affected their child.

The parents who used their phones, on average, had less *mind-minded* thinking about their young children; they were more likely to see their child as *difficult* rather than reflecting on the family dynamics that shaped their child's behavior. This suggested 1 of 2 things: Either parents who felt mentally distant from their kids used technology during family times—possibly as an avoidance strategy—or the regular displacement of mealtime conversations made it harder for parents to look under the hood of what their child was experiencing.

In fact, in a detailed analysis of the same mealtimes published in 2022, we found that for every 5-second interval that parents texted or scrolled on a mobile device, parent talking decreased 52%, child talking decreased 38%, and parents were more than twice as likely to ignore a child's bid for attention. When this is repeated over and over, it makes sense that parents might be less aware of how their child is thinking or feeling.

School Years

Around first grade, many kids start to perceive that they are different from other children. This might be based on appearance (she wears glasses, but I don't) or preferences (he likes basketball, and I like soccer) but also starts to be based on abilities (he's reading chapter books already, and I'm still sounding out words). In my (Jenny) experience, some children with attention-deficit/hyperactivity disorder (ADHD) or learning disabilities start to feel self-conscious about their differences in elementary school and sometimes say things like "I'm stupid," which can be very upsetting for parents to hear. This type of negative self-perception can last through high school if ADHD or learning disabilities aren't effectively managed. Getting negative feedback from teachers and principals also reinforces this; kids who are suspended for acting out often develop a sense that "school can't handle me" or "I can't handle school."

When children don't like school or homework, video games or TV often becomes a preferred activity. Digital games and favorite shows provide satisfaction, a sense of mastery, and a comfort zone that many of our patients seek out after a stressful school day. When there aren't clear time limits, video games can become an avoidance tactic that gets in the way of completing homework (who wants to do a boring math worksheet when there's a highly rewarding go-kart race or battle royale to play?). A 2019 meta-analysis of 58 different studies published in *JAMA Pediatrics* found that more daily time spent on TV and video games, in particular, was associated with lower school performance.

What can you do?

- Have consistent time limits on TV, devices, and video games after school, or limit video games to weekends only. Some studies suggest that when video gaming goes above 2 or more hours per day, child and teen well-being decreases, so choose a similar time limit that fits into your family schedule.
- Manage ADHD or learning differences early to help children's sense of self stay positive around school. Don't wait until fourth or fifth grade. Work with the school on an Individualized Education Program (IEP), 504 plan, and accommodations that help the child handle their emotions in school, make more

progress in the academic tasks that don't come naturally to them, and build a positive friend group.

- Find offline areas of strength and nourish them. This could be music, athletics, art, or other hands-on activities. For my (Jenny) patients, these have included basketball, playing piano, repairing cars, or being a community helper (eg, shoveling snow or mowing lawns for neighbors).
- Don't simply avoid challenges. Kids who are *demand avoidant* (a behavioral profile in which kids have intense resistance to everyday demands like chores or transitions) can push back against challenges. It's fear of discomfort or failure that drives their avoidance (and their preference for low-friction online spaces like video games). However, it's important not to avoid all challenges with these sensitive kids. Being able to manage small stresses and take age-appropriate risks (see Chapter 15) is essential to their sense of self-efficacy.
- Help your children understand that there are all kinds of minds. We all bring strengths and challenges to our lives—it's *understanding yourself* and *working with your unique strengths and challenges* that lets you be successful.

Tech Corner | **What About Digital Play?**

Children explore a lot of different personas and perspectives during imaginative play, and this helps refine their sense of who they are and what they are good at. For older children and teens, playing board games and strategy games helps them learn how to be a good winner and loser. Playing team sports and music together helps kids learn to co-regulate with each other—something that happens when kids pay attention to each other's body language, adapt their behavior to suit what their teammates are doing, and collaborate rather than compete. All types of play involve self-regulation, which means that kids decide when to start and stop, which rules to follow, and how to handle emotions when unexpected things happen.

A lot of these aspects of play can happen on a well-designed digital game (other than the fact that kids are not in the same physical space together). Here are a few red flags that indicate a digital experience is *not* supporting play.

- **Only watching other people play.** One of the most popular genres on YouTube is watching other people play video games or unbox and play with toys. However, this is just vicarious and often mesmerizing and doesn't carry the benefits of play.

  What you can do. If you don't want your child watching this type of content, avoid YouTube altogether or closely manage which channels they watch. If you're OK with your child occasionally watching this type of content, watch along to make sure the YouTuber isn't rude or inappropriate. Also, build on the ideas they see in the video. For example, if they see a family playing "the floor is lava" in a video, try playing that together; if they watch a YouTuber build something cool in *Minecraft*, encourage them to try building and expanding on it.

- **Commercialized play.** In many free online games, our (Jenny) research has found that the whole gameplay experience can consist of accruing in-game currency, spending it, and showing off your new in-game items. These types of repetitive experiences don't involve much strategy or creativity, and our research team called it *consumer grooming*—teaching kids to overfocus on making and spending money. Many of these games also have components similar to those of gambling, which can normalize gambling (see Chapter 15) and lead to more problematic media habits (see Chapter 14).

  What you can do. Work with your kids to save up to purchase games that don't have in-game purchases but feature more creativity or strategy. Saving up could include having daily chores and a small weekly allowance so that they learn the value of the real money they used to purchase the game. Take a break from free games that have more of a commercialized focus and replace them with board games that involve financial concepts such as *Monopoly*, *Dominion*, *Settlers of Catan*, or *Splendor*.

- **Playing with strangers and AI.** Playing with friends builds relationships, trust, and teamwork. Playing with strangers can open kids up to harassment or exploitation, and AI bots embedded in video games are an empty form of companionship.

  What you can do. If your child has friends who could join a multiplayer video game at the same time, arrange this at a predictable time of day or week. Become your child's gaming buddy or look for in-person board game or trading card game opportunities in your neighborhood. Many schools have after-school clubs for *Magic: The Gathering*, *Dungeons & Dragons*, chess, LEGO, or *Pokémon Go*.

- **Dehumanizing activities.** Video games that focus on domination, violence, or gore or involve stereotypes can shape child and teen values in ways that run contrary to your family's norms.

  What you can do. Find other ways your child or teen can feel mastery or get out aggressive energy. This could be through physical activities that allow them to measure their progress over time (eg, running times, martial arts belt colors). Also look for reasons that they might be feeling small, such as bullying.

Teen Years

Friends become an important mirror for sense of self during the teen years. These years are dominated by the questions Who am I? What matters to me? What am I good at?—and peer feedback, offline and online, is a major way that these questions get answered. As parents, it's exciting to watch when this is going well, as our kids gravitate toward activities or academics that click with them. But it can be painful to watch when it's not going well, and teens feel lost, floating around to see what grabs their attention or avoiding engaging in things that seem too hard or boring. Spending time in low-friction or anonymous online spaces can seem safer to them than putting themselves out there.

When teens find the online world more appealing than their offline world, it helps to take a multilevel approach.

- Address any school support needs, as we described in the School Years section earlier in this chapter.
- Figure out what in-person friend or community activities feel doable to them, and support them to schedule those.
- Try to spend more quality family time with your teen or support them in spending time with another trusted adult such as an aunt, uncle, or teacher who connects with them. You can start small, with brief moments of connection on a walk or car ride or something you know your teen finds interesting (eg, cooking, puzzles, shopping).
- Think about therapy to build insight into their sense of self and how depressed or anxious thoughts or moods might be affecting their self-perception.

Practical Takeaway | **Balancing Privacy and Monitoring**

Teens naturally need (and want!) more privacy as they get older. They want their bedroom door closed and sometimes prefer to talk things over with their friends rather than their parents. This increased need for privacy both is developmentally appropriate—they can handle more on their own and don't need a parent intervening all the time—and allows them space to understand their developing self. It can feel like a rejection to parents, so it's an important time to adjust your scaffolding to have a lighter touch, based upon what you think your unique teen is ready for. However, it's still important to monitor and communicate.

Just like you still need to know whose house they are going to and whom they are hanging out with, you will need to monitor their online experiences too. How can you do this without being too invasive?

- Make sure they are aware if you track their location through a watch or device. Location tracking should be used as a check-in that can allow more freedom. For example, when our teenagers first got their licenses, it was reassuring to use location tracking to check that they had arrived at their destination. Don't use it as constant surveillance tactic.
- Be aware that parental controls and safety settings are a bare minimum. Think of the online world as the biggest Wild West neighborhood you could possibly let them explore. Safety settings keep them out of the bars, peep shows, and dark alleys, but they can still get into get into trouble on the main thoroughfares.
- Start with stricter oversight of the apps and games that they download. You can loosen the reins if you see your child showing more self-control and maturity, but continue to monitor.
- Couple parental controls with regular conversations. The most detailed parental monitoring apps can never tell you how your child is feeling.
- Remember to ask them what's going well, and tell them when they are doing a great job. I (Megan) led a teen panel at a community event and asked the teens about how they received positive feedback on their technology behaviors from their parents, and all the teens on the panel said they had never experienced that. It was a great reminder that just like we should tell teens they are doing a great job with their homework, their chores, or their sports, we should also learn about how well they manage their tech use and offer them positive feedback.

Teenage Sense of Self and the Digital World

Building a healthy sense of self while interacting with the digital world involves positive interactions with family (see Chapter 1), peers (see Chapter 2), and parasocial relationships (see Chapter 3), but here we mostly focus on how the self is expressed and experienced online.

Self-Expression

Since the internet was invented, people have found it to be an effective way to reach a lot of people with their thoughts. Early versions included blogs or online diaries where you could narrate your experiences or share your niche interests and skills.

Now social media is the venue for sharing your voice. One of my (Jenny) patients, a middle schooler with autism, liked posting her anime drawings on social media and receiving feedback from other artists. Studies have found that authentic self-expression on social media can support teens' sense of self in that teens can document some of their experiences and creativity, get feedback, and see their evolution of interests over time.

How can you guide your teen on *how much* to share about themselves? This can be a tricky balance of protecting privacy while also enjoying self-expression.

- If your teen is interested in sharing content with other like-minded teens, encourage them to create a private group on a social media platform where they can share posts and ideas. This still allows them to keep their profile private and avoid being contacted by strangers.
- There are ways to engage in creative self-expression while still protecting key aspects of one's identity. Information to keep private includes school name or mascot, home address, any personal identification information, and neighborhood name. Some teens use nicknames or shorten their names for themselves or family members.
- Avoiding location sharing or being careful with tagging location on pictures can also help maintain privacy.

A Social Media Do-Over

I (Megan) have had several patients talk to me about their approach of having a social media do-over. Typically, this involves reviewing existing social media profiles and either deleting old content or deleting the entire profile. These actions may be motivated by a life transition, such as going from high school to college or joining the military. These transitions may lead a teen to want to clean up their online presence, particularly if they feel like they have outgrown aspects of how they used to share information about themselves. Maybe they used to have an entire profile dedicated to their collection of baseball cards, but that's not really their thing anymore. Maybe they have changed their appearance with different hair, or they have grown a lot taller or dress differently. These are typical ways that teens can review, process, and shape their online presence to ensure it feels comfortable to them.

Selfies

Before the front-facing camera was invented, people had to have their picture taken by other people (say cheese!). Before digital cameras, you usually only took one picture, and you got what you got! Jenny and I recall a few gems of photos taken during our tween and teen years in the '80s and '90s—eyes partially closed or with a big red glare, braces sparkling. Photos could make you humble! You also had to be choosy because camera film cost a lot, and it took days to weeks to have it developed. There was no way our parents would allow us to buy rolls and rolls of camera film and pay to have them developed just to get the best, cutest, or funniest photo of ourselves possible.

For today's youth, photos are a different experience. Smartphone cameras have a lot of advantages—how cool is it that you can quickly record a special moment or take a quick photo of something beautiful that you'd like to remember? But when your child or teen receives their first phone or tablet capable of taking photos, there are a few things to review with them before they get going.

One area to review is settings. On some phones or tablets, you can disable the camera app if you don't want your child to get into the habit of photographing everything or themselves. On the other hand, many children use the camera app creatively. As long as they can't post photos and videos online, it is often nice to see what objects they choose to take photos of and how they see the world through a camera lens. I (Megan) remember my son loving the camera filters on our tablet, and I found dozens (maybe hundreds) of photos of our cats as he experimented with light, color, backgrounds, and image distortion. Good thing we have tolerant cats!

Privacy is also an important topic. It may sound obvious, but it is worth ensuring your child knows that selfies are inherently images of themselves. Some may be goofy or pretty or showing different expressions or blurry. But they are all selfies and should be shared carefully and intentionally, with appropriate privacy settings, if shared in online spaces.

Safety while taking selfies is also something to touch on with your child. Selfies should not be taken while driving. Selfies should also be avoided in situations that may pose safety risks, such as biking, skateboarding, or walking someplace where they could be hit by a moving vehicle. Furthermore, taking selfies in high-risk locations, such as at dangerous heights or in unsafe waters, is something to talk to your kids about, since those settings can feel exciting and teens may want to document their location. Overall, ensure your kids don't put themselves at risk while taking a selfie.

Definition

Several years ago, a viral challenge emerged called **rooftopping** in which people would gain access to tall urban buildings, often illegally, to take artistic photos and selfies. This was a very high-risk activity that led to deaths and injuries. (For more on other viral challenges, see Chapter 15 on risky behaviors.)

Conversation Tips | **Reflecting on Selfies**

- Talk to your kids about how it felt if you grew up in a time before selfies were popular and what you liked or didn't like about old-school photos.
- Help your child understand that kids and teens who fixate on selfies often edit them or use beautifying filters to make themselves look better and that this is linked with lower self-esteem. This might surprise them, since the kids with perfect-looking selfies online probably come across as more confident, and they may not realize that those kids could actually feel pretty small inside.
- Remind them that altered selfies can be a sign that they are comparing their appearance to an unrealistic ideal or falsely deleting parts of themselves (acne, frizzy hair) that they are too critical about. If you do notice them critically editing selfies, use a few of the conversation approaches from Chapter 12.
- Support their digital literacy about posting selfies online. Does this change how people value them versus objectify them? Does it lead to social comparison? Does it convey all the cool things about them that can't be captured in a photo?

Commodification of Self

It's common to hear about people having a *personal brand* to sell to others, whether it be to get a job, increase their *social capital* (also called *clout*), or influence what others think or do.

However, having a branded online persona can be problematic for adults as well as teens because it can create distance between the product people see online versus that person's true inner experience. Teens and adults with a weaker sense of self might find it more satisfying and easier to interpret the quantified approval of the "product" they post online—counting likes, followers, and shares—compared with the uncertainty that they feel as a natural part of life and human relationships.

Teens also deserve the opportunity to shift and try out different versions of themselves while they explore their emerging identity. Having a commodified online brand can restrict this type of natural exploration.

For example, a teenage patient of mine (Megan) was a talented artist who had a moderate online following. When she reached a certain number of followers on social media, the platform asked her if she would like to monetize and earn ad dollars when people watched her videos. This created pressure to keep performing and posting content about her art, even though, personally, she was ready to move on to other interests.

Also, research shows that many content creators will adapt their content to the algorithm, meaning that they create more of whatever is trending and getting clicks. I (Jenny) have observed this in my YouTube research: Teen influencers hop to whatever viral challenge or trend receives and attracts the most attention, which is not helpful for a stable sense of self. Think about it: When your environment and community are predictable, you can be a stable version of yourself every day. You show up at school, see the same teachers and classmates, and can bring your same self to those interactions. When your context is constantly shifting, like with a virtual world that sometimes adores you and sometimes ignores you, you will feel pressure to shift with those rapidly changing tides. This doesn't give teens the opportunity to have a stable inner sense of who they are and what people like about them.

As a sidenote, we recognize that it's a valid question whether teens should be influencers at all. There's a difference between expressing your skills authentically online versus performing online to accrue followers and brand deals. As a 2024 *New York Times* investigation of Instagram teen influencer accounts showed, many of the followers were child predators or left lewd comments. Our advice is that teens generally should have private social media accounts. If they are talented enough to be "discovered" online, they can look for an agent who helps manage their online presence and protects them from unwanted contact.

Personal branding is everywhere online, so it's easy to spot and talk about with teens. Help them see the difference between quantified "likes" versus the positive, but more subtle, feedback they might get from school or friends.

Key Point

Send your kids the message that life is about *enjoying the process* rather than *being a product.*

Online Cultures of Self-Improvement

Teens have a lot of questions about their identity and where they fit in the world, and many influencers act like they have all the answers. One way that influencers cultivate a following, get sponsorships, and sell products (such as cosmetics, hair products, or supplements) is to make promises of self-improvement. It can seem like there is a blurred line between a channel or content creator who is providing helpful advice about mental health, makeup tips, or workout suggestions and a creator who is taking advantage of viewers' insecurities and selling *self-optimization*. The following are some questions you can ask your teen to help them discern that line:

- Do you ever see things online that seem to make promises about looking better, being more successful, or being healthier? How do you know what is worth watching?
- Can you tell when a video is sponsored? Does that change your level of trust in the video or content creator?
- Do you think people need to be optimized? What helps you feel happy in your own skin?

Social media can be a fun-house mirror

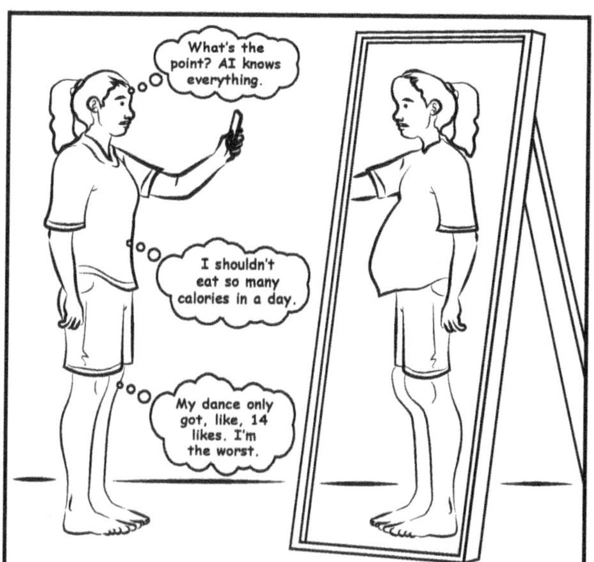
What's the point? AI knows everything.
I shouldn't eat so many calories in a day.
My dance only got, like, 14 likes. I'm the worst.

Tech Corner | **How Data Profiling Affects What We See Online**

Marketing researchers have known for decades how to segment consumers into different categories, study their behavior, and send sales pitches that match their interests and personality. Since mobile devices, social media, and AI were introduced, marketers have much more data about our personal lives, which helps them target us with more precision, whether it be for products or political ideas.

Data profiling also can lead platforms to connect us to others with similar interests when they notice similar patterns in our usage data. This has unfortunately led to political filter bubbles where people only interact with like-minded users. A 2024 study out of the Stanford Internet Observatory found that profiling also led to teen users being recommended to online predators. This is why private accounts are particularly important for young users.

Data profiling also determines what shows up in feeds, which are often labeled in ways such as the For You feed on TikTok. This might send the message to a teen that the recommended content aligns with their self, interests, or identity. Could this shape their interests and norms too, if they get taken down the rabbit hole toward more extreme content? Platforms have called this *preference amplification*, and it could include problems such as the following:

- Concentrating on content about beauty and fitness ⟶ receiving more eating disorder–adjacent content
- Starting with sad content (what some teens call *depression reels* that wallow in negative feelings) ⟶ being recommended self-harm and suicide content (Hundreds of families who are suing social media companies allege that this has happened to their teens.)
- Progressing from gym workout videos ⟶ influencers who focus on masculinity, such as the manosphere, a network of online communities that promote misogyny and aggressive ideas of what

it means to be a man, such as physical dominance and emotional control of women

- Starting with videos about alternative medicine → being recommended influencers who promote anti-vaccine and unproven therapies
- Progressing from videos of your favorite sports team → videos of sports betting or gambling accounts

What can parents do? First, advocate for state or federal laws that prohibit profiling teens by their usage data and engagement-based training of algorithms, which tends to lead to amplification of more extreme content. Second, teach kids and teens about how they are profiled and how this shapes the content and ads they see. Ask questions such as "What do the platforms you use know about you?" Help teens understand that they are more than the ways they are profiled by platforms, which can only measure their demographics, preferences, and where they focus their attention or money. We all have an inner life that is rich and interesting and can never be fully measured by online data.

Connecting the Dots

Adults and children now have digital mirrors in addition to the family, peers, and community that mirror back their sense of self. Sometimes the profit motives of tech companies can create fun house mirrors that warp our sense of self and worth. Parenting around this issue can involve a strong focus on building a rich offline sense of self, while teaching kids about the ways their self can be expressed authentically online.

- **Talk to your kids about it:** What does their favorite platform know about them? Their age, their gender, their favorite things? How is this good or bad? When have tech platforms gotten it wrong?
- **Look at this resource together:** #HalfTheStory is a nonprofit dedicated to improving the next generation's relationship with

technology. Larissa May founded #HalfTheStory after facing her own struggles with social media and now creates resources for youth to have healthier relationships with media. Look at www.halfthestoryproject.com/programs/social-media-u and talk about the idea that "the grass is always greener behind the screen." Does this resonate with your teen? What offline activities help them connect with their inner self?

Chapter 12

BODY IMAGE

What we will cover

- Understanding the components of body image
- Addressing facts and fears about media and body image
- Discussing how you can help your child develop a healthy body image
- What you can do if you are worried about your child's body image

Body image is an important concept that generally starts to develop in early adolescence and is something that can change for everyone throughout their life. The importance of this concept, and the strong evidence linking media to an individual's body image, is why we wanted this concept to have its own chapter. This chapter has cross-references to our chapters on body movement and physical activity (see Chapter 6) and diet and nutrition (see Chapter 7), so we recommend reading through them to see how they affect each other.

What Is Body Image?

Body image is a multidimensional concept made up of 4 components.

1. **Global subjective satisfaction:** How you evaluate your body and your overall assessment of it. Examples may include the following:
   - "I like how tall I am, but I wish I was a little more muscular."
   - "I have a curvy body shape, and that's cool."

- "I look pretty good but could lose a few pounds."
- "I'm so tiny and wish I was bigger and stronger."

Definition

Body image is how we each, as individuals, think and feel about how our body looks. Body image includes our own perceptions of our physical body, as well as our thoughts, beliefs, feelings, and behaviors concerning our physical body.

2. **Affection:** How you feel and the emotions you have about your body. Examples may include the following:
   - "I feel good about my body."
   - "I feel frustrated that I'm not as tall as my brother."
   - "I am happy that I look a lot like my grandpa."
3. **Cognition:** How you think objectively and logically about your appearance and beliefs about the body. Examples may include the following:
   - "I think that if I start track season, I will need to eat a little more to avoid losing weight and make sure I am fueling myself for long runs."
   - "I think if I color my hair then maybe people won't notice that my feet are so big."
4. **Behaviors:** Behaviors that are used to avoid situations in which people can see or are exposed to your body. Examples may include the following:
   - "In winter it is easier for me to dress because I like baggy clothes to hide my belly."
   - "I never change in the locker room because I'm worried people will make fun of my body."

Body image can also be affected positively or negatively by input from one's family or peer group or by ethnic and cultural factors.

Body dissatisfaction is defined as negative thoughts and feelings of a person about their body. It may include negatively evaluating body size, shape, or weight. This usually means the person feels there is a difference between how they think their body looks and what they think of as an ideal body. Rates of body dissatisfaction vary across the world, but in the United States, a study in 2019 in the journal *Clinical Psychological Science* reported that this is estimated to affect 20% to 40% of females and 10% to 30% of males. A 2011 statewide survey of adolescents in California published in the *Journal of the American Academy of Nurse Practitioners* found that 24% of girls and 22% of boys reported body dissatisfaction.

Key Point

Why do body image and body dissatisfaction matter? Dissatisfaction with body image has been linked to poorer self-esteem and increased risk of depression. It has also been linked to poorer dietary quality and eating disorders.

Body Image: Is It All Related to Media?

These days, parents hear a lot about body image in the news and how it may be linked to social media use. This news coverage can lead parents to think that media is the main factor linked to body image and that it is always linked to body dissatisfaction. In this section, we'll address these fears with facts.

Researchers have been doing studies in the area of body image for a long time. What these studies have found is that media is not the only or the main influence on body image. The fact is that there are 3 main factors that influence body image—peers, parents, and media.

Peers

Peer influence on body image typically begins in the preteen years, often between the ages of 10 and 13. Youth who feel accepted by their peers, and are well-connected to at least one peer group, generally have more positive feelings about themselves and their bodies.

There are also some negative influences and behaviors that can lead to body dissatisfaction or affect body image for youth.

- Frequent peer conversations about weight, size, or dieting
- Having peers who are trying to diet or lose weight
- Having peers who are critical about their own, or others', weight or shape
- Hearing peers criticize or tease others about weight or shape

You may be wondering what types of conversations your kids are having with peers about this. The best way to find out is to ask. You can even use this book as your prompt to say, "I was reading a book about how people develop a sense of body image. I learned that peers are an important influence on the development of individual body image, and the way you talk about this topic with your peers is a key part of that. I'm curious, how do you and your friends talk about this topic? Do you hear your friends being overly critical of their bodies or of other people's? Do your friends talk about weight, size, or dieting?"

If they have not been having conversations about these topics, here are a couple of options on how to respond.

- "I'm glad to hear that. I want to keep this topic open, so if you ever have concerns or questions about this, we can talk about it."
- It is OK to share your own experiences if you'd like to round out the conversation, which might be something like "I'm glad to hear that. When I was growing up, it was really common to talk about dieting, and I still remember that those discussions never made me feel good. If you ever have that experience, please know that you can talk to me."

If they are having these conversations, the following are a couple of options of how to respond, keeping in mind that you don't have to fix or solve a bigger situation with just one conversation. You are aiming to open the door to ongoing communication.

- "How do you feel during or after those conversations? Do you have any thoughts or concerns about your own body image?"

- You can share your own experiences while encouraging your child to come to you if they ever want to talk about anything that concerns them.

During the preteen years, your child is likely spending more time with friends, and more time with friends means you aren't there every moment. You may not know if these types of conversations are happening or if your child's peers are engaging in behaviors like dieting. You can weave these questions into conversations with your child in a few ways.

- When watching media that includes a story about dieting or wanting to be a different body shape or size, you can check in on what your child thinks of it, as well as whether they are hearing similar things from others. If you are looking for movies with body positivity, consider *Little Miss Sunshine, Real Women Have Curves, The Full Monty,* and *Hairspray.*
    - You can start with questions such as "What did you think of this story and how they were talking about body shape? Have you seen other stories that are similar in TV or movies?"
    - You can then check in on their peers: "Another way that we hear opinions and thoughts on body shape and size is from our friends. How do you and your friends talk about body image?"
- You can directly check in on how things are going with your child's friends. Asking what they like to do together is one way to start the conversation on a topic not related to body image. Then you can shift the conversation. There are several ways to do this.
    - Share a book with them that talks about teen body image and how important it is to overall health (you can search for lists of these books online). Let your child know you are curious about how they and their friends talk about this topic, as you know their friends are really important to them.
    - You could also consider sharing a story from your own experience: "I have a friend who talks a lot about her latest diet. I feel bad that she has had such struggles with how she sees her weight and body because I really care about her and want her to feel happy about herself. Do you have any friends

like that?" An alternative approach could be "I have a friend who really wants to build more muscle and is often showing me social media posts of what he thinks he should look like. I really care about him and wish he felt good about how his body looks."

Practical Takeaway | **Managing Peer Influences**

I (Megan) remember when a patient told me about watching an awards show with her friend the night before. The show featured a celebrity red carpet, where famous people would walk along it in front of the cameras. She shared that her friend was very critical about some of the attendees, noting their dresses were ugly or they looked fat in their outfit or commenting on whether they had gained or lost weight. She shared that it got her thinking about what she would look like in some of the dresses and worried about what her friend thought of her appearance. She also mentioned that she didn't like to go to her friend's house to hang out because her friend's parents were often critical of what her friend wore or would tease them about gaining weight when snacking. As a pediatrician, I found that this was a situation in which I could really see the connection between how peers can influence body image and how much teens learn from their parents about body image. This experience also demonstrated how you as a parent can have a huge positive influence on body image not only for your own child but also for their friends.

Parents

Parent influence on body image is a critical aspect throughout a child's life. Parents who are warm, affectionate, and emotionally available create an environment around a child that tends to help youth feel comfortable with themselves and feel safe and healthy. Research studies have found that young adolescents who describe their parents as warm and nurturing are more likely to have positive body image than adolescents who described

> **Key Point**
>
> What if you as a parent are in a situation where you need to lose weight for your health? It is OK to acknowledge with your family that you have concerns about your body size or health and that you plan to make changes in your diet or exercise patterns. This framing teaches your child that you are focused on the health of your body and that you are going to make changes to become healthier. Don't bring it up every day or at every meal. Your child may have questions if they are curious, and you can answer those and provide reinforcement that sometimes people need to change their diet or movement patterns to be healthier. This approach teaches your child that we can make changes in our behavior to keep ourselves healthy without doing so in a way that focuses on negative body image.

their parents as more harsh, critical, or emotionally unavailable. The positive effect of having warm and supportive parents on youth body image is also long-lasting. Research studies have found that youth with positive and supportive parents have more consistent body image satisfaction over their childhood and into adulthood.

Studies have also found that when parents are critical of their child's bodies, or their own bodies, it can have a negative effect on their child's body image. Being critical of one's own body as a parent typically means frequently talking about dieting or being on diets or sharing negative feelings about one's own body image. These behaviors can all have a direct effect on children. Being critical of one's body in front of children teaches them that a body is something to be evaluated, scrutinized, and criticized publicly. Talking about and engaging with dieting can teach children that this is normal behavior for any person, and some children will even try dieting at a young age, just like their parents, if they perceive this is what they are supposed to be doing. These critical approaches to one's body are grounded in body dissatisfaction and teach children that body dissatisfaction is normal.

When parents are critical of their children's weight, shape, eating patterns, or size, it is also associated with negative body image. This does not just include direct critical comments but can also include joking and teasing.

Body Image and Media

So how exactly does media affect body image? There have been many studies of how media can influence body image.

Idealized Body Image

Media can present idealized bodies that are not achievable by most humans. Even before photoshopping, airbrushing, and filters, media celebrated bodies that were impossibly tall, thin, muscular, or toned. These images often led to comparisons with one's own body and being overly critical about it.

It is important to realize that idealized body image issues and media were present long before social media emerged. Depending on your age and where you grew up, you may have been exposed to idealized body image media content growing up. The research shows how powerful these forms of media were on influencing adolescent thoughts and behaviors. For example, a 1999 research study in the journal *Pediatrics* surveyed girls in the 5th through the 12th grades about influences on body image. It found that 69% of the girls reported that magazine pictures influenced their idea of the perfect body shape and that 46% wanted to lose weight because of magazine pictures. It also found that there was a positive relationship between the *frequency* of reading fashion magazines and the likelihood of having tried to diet.

A study in 2000 in the *Journal of Communication* measured exposure to 4 types of media.

1. Body-improvement media content, such as magazine articles encouraging readers to "lose weight fast!"
2. Thin-ideal TV and magazines that promoted thin as the ideal body type
3. *Fat-character* TV (a term the researchers proposed—we don't like it) that involved an overweight character in a TV show who was a focus of teasing and jokes
4. Sports magazines

The study found that exposure to thin-ideal magazines, fat-character TV, and sports magazines predicted eating disorder symptoms for female viewers and that exposure to fat-character TV predicted body dissatisfaction for male viewers. This study includes several types of body image–related content and shows how powerful that content can be in making us feel bad about how we look.

Social media can make these existing patterns and trends even worse. Many images on social media are altered, making the body type seem even more desired or ideal despite its alterations. Teens may not always know which images are real and which are altered, but their takeaway may still be that they should look like that model or athlete. The use of AI and other tools in technology add to this problem, as they can create images not based in real life and present wildly unattainable body shapes.

It's important to remember that body image is not just an issue for female adolescents. A 2025 report from Common Sense Media found that 91% of 11- to 17-year-old adolescent males were exposed to body image or appearance content online; 75% saw content about being muscular. Other content included dressing a specific way (47%), being tall (43%), having clear skin (38%), or having a certain jawline (25%). Teens with higher exposure to these types of content were 4 times more likely to say they felt the need to change themselves.

A positive aspect of social media is that youth can find representations of people who look like them, which was something that was lacking in many older types of broadcast media. Finding people on social media who look like you, or have your background or identity, can create a powerful sense of belonging. Social media platforms can play a role in promoting this. For example, in 2024 the social media site Pinterest started letting users choose their preferred body size for fashion posts to reduce the negative body comparison that can result when beauty or fashion is always about thin bodies. On the other hand, if the role model your child finds on social media also has a thin-ideal body, or promotes dieting, that may lead to that person being an even more powerful and relevant influence on your child.

When a youth views thin-ideal or unhealthy body images on social media, that behavior itself can affect a youth's social media algorithm, which means that they receive even more content like this going forward. In research studies such as the 1999 *Pediatrics* study mentioned earlier in this section, the *frequency* of exposure to body image content had an additive effect on teens. The more content they saw in media about a thin-ideal body image, the more likely it was that they would try to diet to attain that body type. Social media functionality itself can increase the frequency of delivering this type of content if your child has viewed it previously. This inundation of idealized body content, coupled with diet and beauty tips, branded product promises, or calls for self-improvement, has a powerful and additive influence over time.

Fat-Shaming

Another unfortunate way that youth can experience negative body image content on social media is through content that engages in *fat-shaming.*

This concept is similar to the *Journal of Communication* research study described in the Idealized Body Image section earlier in this chapter that had a fat character as a source of comedy. Fat-shaming can happen in all corners of the internet and social media. It can be the focus of a video, an image, or a post. It can also show up in comments on someone else's video, image, or post. These comments can be incredibly rude, harsh, and cruel.

> **Definition**
>
> **Fat-shaming** is humiliating someone who is perceived as overweight by mocking or giving critical comments about their size.

Fat-shaming can contribute to unhealthy behavior and outcomes. A 2019 summary article in the *Canadian Medical Association Journal* presented outcomes from a national summit on the topic of obesity. The author states that fat-shaming can lead to a unique form of stress, which triggers the hormone cortisol, as well as embarrassment and shame. The combination of higher cortisol, less self-control due to embarrassment, and shame can lead to an increased risk of binge eating. Findings from the summit concluded that the more people were exposed to fat-shaming, including weight bias and discrimination, the more likely they were to gain weight and have obesity. Fat-shaming has also been linked to mental health problems including depression, anxiety, and low self-esteem.

Tech Corner | **How Designs Influence Body Image**

Filters on social media can have *beautification* designs, such as smoothing out skin appearance, changing eye color or cheekbone shape, or even showing what you would look like after plastic surgery (eg, lip filler). Research has shown that use of these beautification filters, or overediting selfies with filters, is linked with lower self-esteem in teens. It's important to talk about these filters with teens, why they are not realistic (or even attractive a lot of the time), and how to love your own face or body.

Algorithmic feeds can recommend celebrity or beauty-related posts that contribute to negative social comparison (the feeling of being "less than") in teens. Released in whistleblower documents, a survey of more than 50,000 users at Instagram found that negative comparison was driven more by top celebrity accounts, which appeared in teen girls' feeds 5 times as often as friends' posts.

Profiling of teens on social media can lead to them being recommended appearance-related content—simply because it is trending with other teens their age or of the same gender. In the 2025 Common Sense Media report about boys' exposure to masculinity content, two-thirds of boys reported that the content showed up in their feed *without* even searching for it.

Female *and* male characters in video games can often have unrealistic body dimensions (eg, Lara Croft from *Tomb Raider*). Try to find video games with more positive body portrayals, but know that it's difficult to avoid all extreme depictions of bodies in our culture (superhero comics have them too). That's why it's important to talk and build critical thinking skills about how our culture places value on appearance and body shape (see suggestions on pages 244–246) while helping kids and teens love themselves.

Thin Shaming

A similar issue is *thin shaming*. Thin shaming also calls out someone's body shape in a negative way. It exposes the person to the feeling of being stared at, judged, and evaluated. It may hinder someone's progress if they are struggling with disordered eating or medical issues.

> **Definition**
>
> **Thin shaming** is criticizing or making negative comments about people being too thin, often using a phrase such as "Eat a sandwich" or calling people names. It is different from fat-shaming because it does not carry the same systemic discrimination, but it does negatively affect body image and mental health.

Body Positivity

Youth can find the positive side of body image through content focused on *body positivity*.

This movement has had a positive effect on driving new marketing campaigns. One you may have seen was from a soap brand that included images of women of all shapes, sizes, and skin colors in their advertisements and commercials. By searching for body positive attributes or traits, your child can influence the algorithm to send more of this type of content to them. Body positivity content can be found through keywords and

> **Definition**
>
> **Body positivity** is a movement to accept bodies of all sizes and types. It lifts up and celebrates bodies regardless of size, shape, or appearance.

hashtags such as #bodyacceptance, #BoPo, and #bodypositivity. Other keywords and hashtags can help direct teens to supportive communities of interest, such as #inclusivefashion for teens who love clothing, #edrecovery for teens recovering from disordered eating, and #effyourbeautystandards for a teen with a rebellious streak.

Key Point

As your teen finds creators they like, encourage them to follow them so that this type of content shows up more frequently on their social media feed. You can also encourage them to mute, unfollow, or unfriend accounts that leave them feeling critical or negative about themselves or jealous of others.

Research Corner | **The Effects of Body Positivity**

Body positivity is a relatively new concept, but research supports that this framework and its application have positive effects.

- A 2015 study found that benefits of a body positivity framework include behaviors that promote self-care, respect for personal needs, and avoiding "exhausting dietary behaviors."
- A 2020 study explored how body positive content affects mood and body image in real time. By sending brief surveys at random points during the day to older adolescents, they found that seeing body positive messages improved mood and body image.
- A 2025 study found that watching short-form videos about body positivity was associated with improved body satisfaction for both male and female participants.

How You Can Help Your Child Have a Positive Body Image

As parents or caregivers, you have a direct role in helping to shape your child's body image. Studies that examine family factors that help kids develop a healthy body image can inform the ways that parents should and should not communicate about body image. Here are some key dos and don'ts.

Dos

In thinking about ways to communicate with your child to support a healthy body image, we'd like to encourage you to use the *3Fs—fabulous* acceptance, *functions* and what your body can do, and *finding* things you like.

- **Share messages of fabulous acceptance:** Everybody has imperfections and flaws, even models in magazines or weight lifting influencers on social media. As a parent, you can share messages of acceptance with your child.
  - You can share a message about accepting your own body, something like the following: "When I was younger, I used to wish I was taller, but I'm really happy to be in a healthy body…and I look fabulous in heels!"
  - You can also share these messages about your child, such as this: "I know you sometimes wish that your body was smaller. I appreciate you sharing your goals to be like that fitness influencer with me. I want to support you in your goals, and I want to share that I think you look wonderful just the way you are. I love that you have such strength and power in your body, and I hope that you love that about yourself too."
  - If you find yourself watching an awards show with your child, pay attention to how they are talking about celebrities' appearances as they walk the red carpet. If they are critical of people's bodies, you could point out how challenging it must be to walk in those heels and how they are totally rocking it or how brave they must be to walk the carpet in front of all those cameras. You can even simply remind them of how

bodies are beautiful in all shapes, colors, and sizes—and, yes, even in that lavender taffeta dress.

- **Lean into what your body can do and how it functions for you:** Rather than comments about what your body looks like, share comments about how much you appreciate what your body can do. Thinking about your body's functionality and strengths is a great way to help remember all the amazing things our bodies do for us every day to help us work and play and get where we want to go.
  - One example is "Wow, we walked 5 miles together today! How awesome to have bodies that have the endurance to do that!"
  - "You did an amazing job learning that TikTok dance you showed me. I am so impressed you learned it so well after 1 day!"
  - You can also focus on what functions really matter in the activities important to your child: "Buddy, your soccer coach doesn't care whether you have 6-pack abs; he cares that you will be first to the ball and work hard at practice."
- **Find things you like about your body:** You can role model this behavior for your child.
  - Find little ways to share joys about how you look. One example may be "Look at this new shirt I bought. It really brings out the color of my eyes!"
  - Look for ways to share these comments with your child. One example is "That new ring looks so nice on your fingers, as it really shows off how lovely your hands are."
- If your child compares themselves to a celebrity or influencer in the media, you can use various types of messages to support your child as they process differences between media bodies and their own bodies. These include using the following:
  - Acceptance: "Well, he has very big muscles that not every person can achieve. But that doesn't mean that you are not also strong in your own body."
  - Leaning into what your body can do and pivoting from appearance to functioning: "She does look very slim in that outfit. And you look awesome in your running clothes. I really admire your approach to running. I love how you run

to see how far you can go, and it seems like a great way to shake off the stress of school and homework."

- Accepting what your body can't do and finding things you like about your body: "I agree. Her long, straight hair is fantastic. I could straighten my hair in the morning and it would still start to curl back up by evening. But one thing I like about both of us is we have similar eyes, and I think we both look great in our glasses."

The 3Fs Approach to Positive Body Image

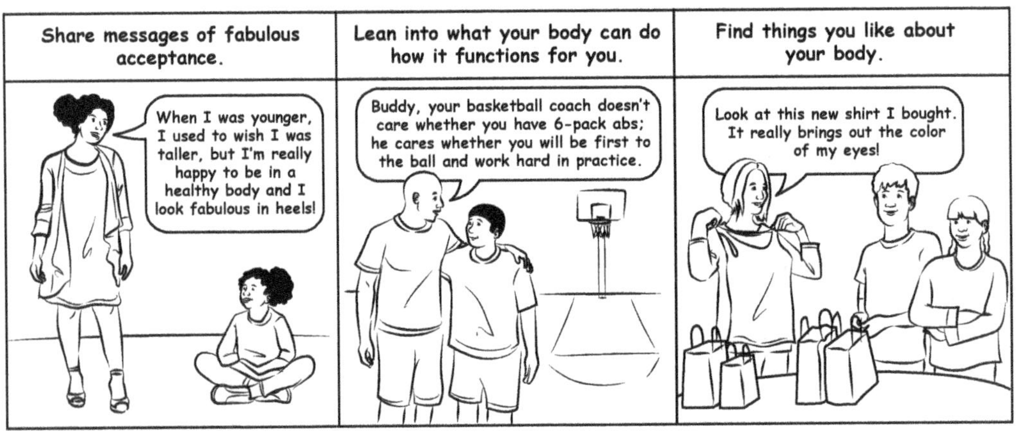
Share messages of fabulous acceptance.
When I was younger, I used to wish I was taller, but I'm really happy to be in a healthy body and I look fabulous in heels!
Lean into what your body can do how it functions for you.
Buddy, your basketball coach doesn't care whether you have 6-pack abs; he cares whether you will be first to the ball and work hard in practice.
Find things you like about your body.
Look at this new shirt I bought. It really brings out the color of my eyes!

Don'ts

The don'ts are tricky, especially if you grew up in a household in which these types of comments or pressure were common. If that was your experience, give yourself some grace. Depending on culture, generational factors, and social pressures, messages about body image are not always healthy or kind. You can be part of changing the narrative around body image and helping your child. If this feels tough for you, or brings up bad memories, find sources of support for yourself. That may include talking with siblings or cousins to process your previous experiences or talking to friends and getting their support. You can even consider therapy so you can let go of your own struggles and embrace your own body image.

A critical behavior to avoid is teasing a person about their weight or food preferences. Although these types of comments can sometimes be intended as harmless or joking, they can have a significant negative effect

Key Point

For adolescents who have existing worries or concerns about their bodies, or who tend to be anxious or worried, negative or teasing types of comments can do harm to their body image.

on a child. I (Megan) remember a patient who described having an uncle who teased her relentlessly about her fifth birthday party when she ate a large piece of cake. "I'm 13 now, and every time I see him [uncle], he asks how big a piece of cake I'm going to have for my birthday. At the holidays, he asked me if I was going to have dinner or just go for cake!"

Media can be part of teasing. Teasing or being critical about a teen's desire to be like people in the media does not help them to change their attitudes and deepens their insecurities about their own bodies. If your child vocalizes that they want to look like an idealized celebrity that they watch on TV or follow on social media, replies such as "Are you joking? That's never going to happen" do not help. Joking and sarcasm such as "Yeah, right, I can totally see *that* happening" are also toxic in this situation. It's better to use one of the 3Fs techniques. For example, you could focus on acceptance, saying something such as "Yes, he is muscular, and I really appreciate how you have a tall and lean build that is awesome for running." You could talk about what their body can do such as "I appreciate that you like how he looks, and I'm reflecting on what a great job you did in your football game last week blocking. I don't know that you could do that so well if you were a lot thinner." Or you could consider things they like about their body: "I get that you like his hair, but your hair is different in texture. What are some things you like about how you look?"

Excessively complimenting or criticizing a person's appearance is another area that can be tricky for family members, especially during adolescence. These types of comments can include positive ones such as "Wow, that outfit looks great on you" to more veiled criticisms such as "That skirt is cute, but a little short, and it makes your legs look big." Keep an eye on these comments, including their tone, the possible intention, and the frequency with which they come up in your household. This is especially critical as your child transitions to adolescence because they are thinking a lot about their developing body and image, and they are paying attention to these types of comments. It can be tempting to look for ways to compliment your child's appearance, especially if they are nervous about it—and doing this from time to time is great. However, having the *main compliments* for your child focused *only* on their appearance can lead to your child seeing themselves as having appearance-related worth.

I (Megan) once heard a thoughtful story from a parent of a patient who had recovered from an eating disorder. The mother shared with me that she had realized her own compliments and interactions with her daughter were quite focused on appearance during her child's early adolescence. She thought her daughter was beautiful and wanted to share that with her by pointing it out frequently. As her daughter recovered from her eating disorder, the mother reflected on how she could best support her daughter in seeing herself as a whole person, beyond her appearance or weight—a person who was kind to her family members, was good at math, liked to read books, wanted to be a dentist, and had a great laugh. She shared this with me:

"I realized I used to do a lot of complimenting her on her outfits or how good she looked. At some point, I realized maybe this wasn't helping. So I tried to compliment her at least 3 times a day and make 2 of them not related to her appearance. It was tricky at first. I ended up just complimenting her on the stuff I thought she should be doing anyhow, like finishing her homework before dinner, or complimenting her on how kind she was to her grandma last weekend. Then I realized I really enjoyed looking for these things she was doing well and sharing them with her. Now I keep doing it out of habit, and it is pretty easy."

"I'm Concerned About My Child's Body Image"

If you are concerned about your child's body image, there may be several reasons for this. You may have heard them make critical comments about themselves. You may also have noticed a pattern of communication in which someone else is sharing comments with your child that are critical, teasing, or mean. There are a few behaviors that may suggest your child is struggling with body image. These include the following:

- **Excessive body checking:** This means looking at, or touching, one's body in front of a mirror to measure size, shape, or appearance.
- **Body avoidance:** This means deliberately avoiding mirrors or activities that draw attention to your body.
- **Dieting:** This refers to changing one's weight, particularly when tied to comments about negative body image or using unhealthy approaches to lose weight.

If you see your child experiencing any of these behaviors, it is worth having a conversation with them.

Ask gently: Find a time to talk calmly with your child about how they feel about their body. You can normalize asking this through approaches such as the following:

"It is normal to sometimes feel a little down about your body or how you look. I'm wondering if you could share how you have been feeling about your body lately."

Or you can share that you are worried and why.

"I've seen you make some comments about your body that are pretty critical lately. It is normal to feel this way at times, but I also want to check in on how you are doing and see how I can help support you."

Observe and listen: Listen to how your child talks about their body, and it may even be helpful to note specific comments to share with them as examples. Listen also to how people around your child talk about bodies—their peers, other family members, maybe even a babysitter. Are there specific voices that may be driving your child's concern? If so, you may want to talk with your child specifically about those comments. You can share ways that your child can shift those conversations by suggesting they say something like this: "Instead of talking about diets, let's talk about the new episode of your favorite TV show that just came out." You can also talk with your child about what may be driving that person's comments; maybe they are worried about how they look, but that doesn't mean your child also needs to take on that worry.

Communicate using the 3Fs strategies: Look for ways to share messages to support your child's own body image. Using the 3Fs, you can find ways to message about fabulous acceptance, what your child's body can do and how well it functions, and finding things you like about your body and encouraging your child to do the same.

Social Media and Eating Disorders

A 2024 study in the *Journal of Eating Disorders* found that having body image issues, combined with spending time on specific types of content on social media, were strong predictors of developing eating disorders. This study shows the risks of engaging in content on social media, specifically content that promotes a thin-ideal body for women or a muscular body shape for men, to youth at risk for eating disorders. This combination of existing risk and exposure to triggering content can greatly increase the risk of developing an eating disorder such as anorexia nervosa or bulimia. This study and others like it highlight how social media, including delivery of image-based and often unrealistic content, combined with the algorithm that continues to deliver similar content, can have a big influence on youth at risk for eating disorders. If you are concerned about your child being at risk for an eating disorder, such as low body image or a focus on dieting and body shape, use the communication approaches described in this chapter and have frequent check-ins on social media content. If you have tried these approaches and their body image is not improving, it may be time to take things to the next level. Schedule a visit with your pediatrician to check in to make sure your child is not having dramatic changes in their weight because of behavioral changes. During that visit, you could ask your pediatrician to talk with your child about body image. Another option is to consider a counselor or mental health provider; there are many out there who have experience in body image concerns.

Connecting the Dots

This chapter has focused on ways to support your child in developing a healthy body image. A key part of parenting on this topic is knowing your child. A child who is more nervous, or worries about how they look, needs more intentionality around how you communicate about this topic. You may need to check in specifically to gauge their feelings about how their body looks. You may need to ask how they and their friends talk about their bodies. You may need to ask your child about the media they are watching or reading and how it makes them feel about how they look. A child who is confident about how they look may mostly need reinforcement of feeling good about themselves. Knowing your child is key to understanding how much work is needed in this area. In knowing your child, remember to know yourself. This topic of body image can be really tough for some parents, so give yourself grace if you find yourself wrestling with some demons from your own past, and make sure to seek out the support you need.

- **Talk to your family about it:** Consider talking to your family about the topics and approaches in this chapter. Over dinner, share the 3 main influences on body image—peers, parents, and media. What do your kids think about those influences in their lives? Consider talking with your co-parent or close friends about the messages you each received about body image growing up and whether those had positive or negative effects on your own body image. How do you each want to communicate with your kids to help them develop a healthy body image?
- **Engage in a challenge:** You may have a family member who often uses communication styles like being critical of people's bodies or teasing people about their bodies—comments that may be unhelpful in fostering and growing your child's body image. This may include a grandparent who makes frequent or borderline inappropriate comments about your child's appearance with them in earshot. This may include an aunt who engages in teasing your child's appearance—or a lot of kids' appearances. It can be a challenge to navigate these uneasy situations, especially if your child is navigating their own uneasiness about their body image.

  Your challenge: Talk to your child about how you feel about that person's comments. This may go something like "I want to share that I often feel uncomfortable when your aunt makes those kinds of comments. We may not be able to change how she thinks or talks, but it is important to me that you know that I do not agree with those comments, and I am sorry that you sometimes hear them. We can both decide to not buy into how she thinks about how people should look."

An additional challenge, should you choose to accept it, would be to have a conversation with that relative. This may be more or less possible depending on your family dynamics and culture. Let's say an aunt comments on one of the cousins who has gained weight. You may consider if there is a way to kindly and clearly share how you feel. These can be tricky conversations and don't always lead to actual change. When talking with her, a helpful approach may be to focus on how you feel, not on who she is. For example, "I feel sad hearing you talk about our cousin this way. I like to think about what a great student he is and how much he helps by playing with the younger kids at these types of gatherings." Even if her behavior does not change, you will know that you have done what you could to shift the conversation away from comments that can negatively affect body image.

Part 4 | **Risky Behaviors**

Chapter 13

VIOLENCE, AGGRESSION, AND HATE SPEECH

What we will cover

- How violence and aggression show up in the media
- How hate speech appears in media
- How you can help limit your child's exposure to violent content and talk about it
- What to do if you are worried about your child's exposure to violent content

As parents, we know that our children will eventually come across types of content we worry about. Violent content can include images, descriptions, or videos showing someone engaging in violent or aggressive behavior, such as pushing, kicking, or hitting another person. It may also include violent or aggressive language such as threats or insults.

In this chapter, we'll unpack each of these areas and how you as a parent can limit your child's exposure and set up conversations to talk about this type of media content to prevent its negative influence.

Definitions

Violence is a particular form of aggression that involves using physical force to harm another person.

Aggression is a broader term for behaviors that are intended to harm another person, which could include through words, relationships, or physical means.

These terms can be used somewhat interchangeably, but whereas all violence involves aggression, not all aggression involves violence.

How Do Violence and Aggression Show Up in the Media?

Violence and *aggression* can show up in many types of media. These media types include TV or movies, video games, music, and social media. Some of these media portrayals are fiction and made-up stories. Other media portrayals are depictions of real-life tragedies and tragic situations that show up in news media or online.

The research on the topic of violence in media goes back decades, spanning across many types of media and showing consistent findings. These findings show that witnessing violent acts in media, whether they are real or fictional, may give children the idea that violence and aggression are normal and acceptable.

It is also thought that seeing a lot of violent content may lead children to act out what they see and hear. In an experiment, preschool children were shown an episode of *Barney* (a prosocial TV show with a big purple dinosaur who sings about friendship), and on the following day they were shown the *Mighty Morphin Power Rangers* (a TV show in which a team fights enemies with martial arts). Immediately after the children watched each video, teachers observed how the children played with each other.

Mimicking violent content

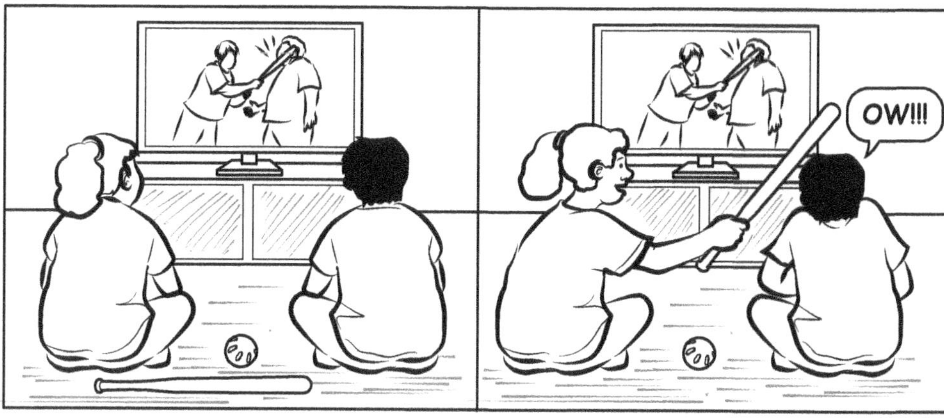

After *Barney*, there was a lot of hugging and singing; after the *Mighty Morphin Power Rangers*, the children's play was full of kicking, wrestling, and other aggression. The study showed that kids are easily primed to copy the world around them.

This risk is even higher if the child sees violence in their life at home or in their community. There are also newer studies suggesting that ongoing exposure to violence, even virtual violence, can trigger mental health conditions such as depression or anxiety.

Media Stories About Bullying

Bullying can occur offline in situations such as schools or neighborhoods. Bullying can also occur online via social media posts or texting and is referred to as *cyberbullying* (see pages 51–52). When cyberbullying first emerged in the early 2000s, researchers studied if this was a different and distinct phenomenon from traditional bullying. After thorough research, the results showed that bullying and cyberbullying are more alike than dissimilar. Research has shown that bullying and cyberbullying often overlap. One 2019 study published in *BMC Public Health* found that 48% of youth involved in cyberbullying also experienced traditional bullying and that 41% of youth involved in traditional bullying also experienced cyberbullying.

Research Corner | **Bullying Prevalence**

Bullying is something that many kids will be exposed to in real life. In 2022, the National Crime Victimization Survey reported that among youth in grades 6 through 12, about 20% reported being bullied during school, and 21% reported cyberbullying. The 2023 Youth Risk Behavior Survey of US youths estimated that about 16% of high school students had experienced cyberbullying in the past year. The Pew Research Center reported in 2022 that nearly half of teens (46%) reported ever experiencing cyberbullying.

As research has progressed, our understanding of roles in a bullying situation and the power of words we use has continued to evolve. We used to refer to someone who engaged in bullying as a *bully*, and the one who was bullied was a *victim*. What we now know is that those labels are extremely powerful and can lock people into thinking of themselves, and others, as just that one thing. It can make it difficult for someone who has been labeled as a bully to be seen as anything else. There has also been the realization that these are not labels but are roles that a kid plays in any given situation. The National Academies of Sciences, Engineering, and Medicine issued a consensus report in 2016, which summarized decades of research and made recommendations, including labeling roles and not people.

In any bullying situation, people can take on one or more roles.

- **Target:** The person or people who are being bullied
- **Perpetrator:** The person doing the bullying
- **Bystander(s):** The person or people watching the bullying occur

Each of these roles can change over time. For example, a bystander may choose to defend the target and thus become a target of bullying themselves. An additional role that is less commonly talked about is that of the *bully-victim*, who is often a child who has been the target of bullying but then takes on the role of perpetrator by bullying others. In research studies, the bully-victim is considered to be a role with many risks and negative consequences. Children who act as bully-victims are at higher risk for negative outcomes involved in both being a target of bullying and being a perpetrator of bullying. Children who are in the role of bully-victims are the most likely to have long-term negative effects from these experiences, including depression, anxiety, and substance use.

So why are we digging into this? It is because media stories about bullying often include a storyline in which the target of bullying finally decides to stand up for themselves and potentially become someone who is a bully-victim. For example, in the movie *A Christmas Story*, Ralphie had finally had enough of being a target of bullying and started a physical fight with the youth who had been bullying him. On the one hand, this action possibly gave viewers a little satisfaction to see the target of bullying finally stand up

Research Corner | **Consequences of Bullying Experiences**

In 2015, I (Megan) was part of a study led by Dr Ellen Selkie that was published in the journal *Cyberpsychology, Behavior, and Social Networking*. We surveyed female college students from multiple colleges across the United States and found that, even among college students, those with past experiences of cyberbullying had increased risks for depression. Participants who had acted as a bully in the past had increased risks of both depression and problematic alcohol use, and participants who had experienced being bully-victims had the highest rates of depression. This study showed the potential for long-term harm to youth involved in cyberbullying, even if they were not in a role as the target of bullying.

for himself, but on the other hand, it highlighted violence and aggression and promoted a story in which a target of bullying emerges as a bully-victim. It also had the potential to teach viewers that starting a fight was the best way to handle bullying, when this is not actually the case. These are very common media stories because, let's face it, in the moment, they can be very satisfying to watch. It can feel good to watch a big mean kid who is bullying others get their due. However, keep in mind that kids are very attuned to these stories and what they teach about social dynamics and power.

Definition

Hate speech is language that targets a group or an individual because of their inherent characteristics such as race, religion, or gender.

Hate Speech in the Media

Hate speech shows up in the media in several places, including social media posts or comment sections, news reports, or online memes. What does this look like? The following are some examples of hate speech:

- **Negative stereotypes:** Media content can push or reinforce negative stereotypes that certain groups are inferior, lazy, or inherently criminal; lack intelligence; or are lesser in some other way.
- **Conspiracy theories:** Media content can create or reinforce conspiracy theories that significant societal problems such as crime, disease, or the breakdown of traditions are the fault of one or more particular groups.
- **Minimizing or denying tragic events:** Media content can minimize or deny tragic events in history, such as the Holocaust or 9/11.

A huge concern with some types of hate speech is that it can be used as a precursor to *atrocity crimes* (which are inhumane acts against people), meaning that hate speech can lead to disinformation that can lead to violent actions being committed.

How to Limit Exposure to Violent Content in the Media

Fortunately, there are some strategies to limit your child's exposure to this type of media.

Tech Corner | **Bullying and Harassment**

According to a 2023 report from the Anti-Defamation League (ADL), 52% of Americans have experienced harassment on social media. The UCLA Initiative to Study Hate surveyed more than 14,000 US tweens and teens and found that 80% of them had encountered hate speech online in the prior month; of that hate speech, 71% was related to race or ethnicity, 72% was related to gender, and 62% was related to religious beliefs. This is a *lot*—and it is distressing to both targets and bystanders.

A few design features contributed to this high prevalence.

- **Anonymity.** When accounts are anonymous, people may think they can get away with inappropriate or unsafe behavior without being caught.
- **Engagement metrics.** These are metrics such as likes, shares, and comments. When people who participate in trolling or harassment realize that they get more engagement when they say extreme things, they may continue this behavior.
- **Use of dog whistles.** Although many social media and gaming platforms try to use machine learning methods to detect and remove aggressive, violent, or hateful speech, they can't always detect the use of metaphors or coded or suggestive language that is aimed at putting down a group of people.
- **Hate speech in AI training data.** If AI chatbots have been trained on data from the internet that includes biases or hate speech, it may get repeated in chatbot interactions.
- **Public online spaces.** These are spaces where youth and adults can interact. For example, industry whistleblowers have reported that virtual reality platforms such as Horizon Worlds allow adults and kids to be in the same game space, and this allows kids to be exposed to hate speech and bullying.

"How Do I Figure Out If Content Includes Violence?"

The US TV rating system includes age-based ratings such as TV-G for general audiences and TV-14 for content that may not be appropriate for children younger than 14. The TV rating system also includes content descriptors, using *V* for violent content and *FV* for fantasy violence (we are not big fans of that terminology). Keep in mind that these ratings are assigned to TV programs by the network that airs the programs, so there are no blanket rules for consistency across networks. It is understandable that there are often a lot of concerns about how accurate, consistent, or helpful this rating system is.

Fortunately, there are other resources you can use to review particular shows, movies, games, or even apps that your child wants to engage with. An excellent one we recommend is the Common Sense Media rating system, which includes all forms of media. Each show, movie, game, or app has had a full review, and the reviewer's name and credentials are listed next to the review so that you know a bit about who created the work. In addition to an overall age recommendation, there is a description of specific types of content within that media, such as violence and scariness; sex, romance, and nudity; drinking, drugs, and smoking; and language level (swearing, slurs, etc). They also highlight positive messages in the story, diverse representation, and positive role models. These reviews can be very helpful to parents as they consider what media is appropriate for their children, to indicate whether it could contain aggression, hate speech, bullying, or domestic violence.

- **For young kids (7 years and younger).** Look at reviews before showing them movies or TV shows. Young children are not yet able to tell the difference between fiction and real life, so violent content can be really scary for kids this age. Younger kids can also get hooked on a show quickly, so, before you show them an initial episode, knowing what language is used, the level of violence, and other aspects is incredibly helpful so you can make an informed decision about whether or not the movie or TV show is appropriate for your child. If you are not sure, watch an initial episode together to check it out.
- **For older kids (8–12 years).** This is a great age to show your kids the review website and ask them to be part of the vetting

before starting to watch a show or play a video game. I (Megan) remember a specific situation when my son was about 10. It was family movie night and my son's turn to pick. At the end of dinner, he excitedly shared, "I already looked [the movie] up, and it is for ages 8+ and here are the reviews on content!" It was great to see him taking charge of picking a movie and looking at the background to make sure it was appropriate for age and content. During this age range, it is pretty likely that your child will have some exposure to violent or aggressive content through media, either at home or at a friend's or family member's home. Setting limits is tough as your child builds more independence, so a key strategy is to talk with your kids about *why* you want to limit their exposure to violent content. You can share that this type of content can make it seem normal to act in violent ways or can lead to feeling more aggression after watching. Help your child consider any connections between what they watch and how they feel so that they can begin to build skills in processing what they see and managing their own emotions and perspectives about what is normal.

- **For teens (13 years and older).** Teens can also be engaged via content from reviews. If they have younger siblings, they can help look up potential family movies to make sure they are appropriate for younger siblings. For parents, these reviews can open opportunities for discussion by looking at the content information for areas you may want to talk about with your teens after the movie. If the movie includes violence, be ready to ask about how it made you both feel watching it. If the movie has positive role models, highlight those characters and talk with your teen about what they liked or found interesting. At these ages, it is very important to ask questions more than to give advice or input. Ask what your teen likes about a movie or show and how they feel about the violent parts, and really listen to their responses. Ask follow-up questions and show you are interested in what they think. This approach helps teens feel heard and helps them develop their own critical thinking skills related to the media they engage with regularly.

Practical Takeaway | **How Old Are You?**

If your teen uses social media, it's crucial that they be honest about their age. Most social media companies now have content filters that are supposed to keep violent, mature, and inappropriate content out of teens' feeds. However, independent investigations of teen accounts have still found that upsetting or unhealthy content gets through these filters. Therefore, it's important to talk with your teen about what is being recommended to them and how to block, report, or downvote violent and hateful content. If your teen set up their social media account with a false age, encourage them to change it to their actual age so that they can get built-in content protections.

"How Do I Figure Out Settings and Controls to Avoid Violent Content?"

There are ways to use settings on your devices or platforms to limit content. Most modern TVs have a V-chip that works with the TV parent guidelines and ratings. You can then set your TV to avoid programs that have certain ratings, such as TV-MA (for mature audiences only). Each TV's V-chip works differently, so it can take a little sleuthing to figure it out. Some TVs have on-screen menu options that include parental settings. If you need help navigating the options, consult the TV instructional guide or the TV company's website.

There are also parental control options on most cable or satellite systems if you use those, as well as within streaming services. On cable TV, most often you can use your remote menu button to find settings. Within the settings, there is a section on parental controls. Most companies have you set a PIN that locks in your selections, so make sure to choose one that your clever kids won't be able to guess. Within those settings, you can also often choose to block certain channels or set blocking for TV or movies based on their ratings. Similar to V-chips, each of these has a slightly different approach to set up the limitations, so a little detective work is often needed. And for many devices, you'll need to establish settings for each device.

For streaming services, you can typically find a section describing parental controls from the main settings menu. Similar to what you would do with cable TV, you create a PIN and restrict types of content. For some streaming services, you can also set limits on time watching in a setting. These settings will affect all devices that use that streaming account.

One thing to keep in mind is that kids, some more than others, are often super tech-savvy people. If you can search online how to set up TV settings to block content, chances are that they can do the same to remove the settings. Kids are endlessly inventive at getting around blocking software and similar programs. This is why blocking alone, without parental communication about why the content is blocked or what concerns you have about the content, is unlikely to be successful in preventing your child from viewing that type of content. Doing the work of communicating about your concerns about media content, such as violence or aggression, can help your child understand your approach, and these conversations can foster trust and respect. This makes the approach feel more like a family approach and overall rule and less like a challenge to the child to figure out how to hack the system. Talk with your kids about the settings you selected and why, and revisit this on at least a yearly basis to see how the settings are working.

As your kids get older, you can involve them more in the choices about what settings to have. I (Megan) had a patient in clinic once who had pretty serious anxiety, and he noticed it worsened when he saw content with fighting or violence. He worked with his dad to set their streaming services to block any content labeled as having violence. That way, when his friends were over and they looked for movies, they didn't see those as options, and he didn't have to try to negotiate avoiding it around friends.

"What If Another Family Member Such as My Co-Parent Loves Action Movies That Have a Lot of Violence?"

In reality, many people enjoy violent media content or don't see an issue with it. When Netflix released the show *Squid Game*, a show with high levels of violence, more than 100 million people watched it. Why did they watch? In 2021, Dr Simon McCarthy-Jones at Trinity College Dublin, a psychologist and neuroscientist, described a couple reasons why some people are drawn to violence in media. First, some people want new and intense experiences in their lives. These are the people we may refer to as *thrill seekers*. For these

Practical Takeaway | **Limiting Exposure to Real-World Violence**

When something scary or tragic happens in the world, it is often on the news 24-7 and appears in everyone's social media feeds. It can be hard to look away, either because of frightening or gripping images or because you want to know what is going on. But intense exposure to real-life violent events can cause children and teens to have anxiety, irritability, trouble sleeping, or physical symptoms like headaches. Children are naturally egocentric, meaning they often worry that similar terrible things will happen to them or their family.

We recommend the following:

- Don't have the TV or radio on constantly. Check intentionally for updates, ideally with kids out of the room, and then turn it off.
- Make sure your teens take more breaks from social media after a violent news event.
- Look for resources from the American Academy of Pediatrics, American Psychological Association, or Common Sense Media on how to talk to kids about what is going on. These resources usually provide helpful explanations that give kids a sense of security and safety.
- Share with your kids, if it seems appropriate, any news reports you can find about the people who are helping solve the problem. You can watch together or talk about the inspirational stories you discovered. As Mister Rogers said, "Look for the helpers."

folks, violent media may provide a jolt of adrenaline and make them feel intense feelings. Second, some people who may enjoy this content are people who are very nervous. These people also feel intense emotions from watching content that is scary or violent, but those feelings are typically anxiety or fear. They may watch this content to try to learn from it. They may feel that exposure to this content will reduce their nervousness if something like that were ever to happen to them. These folks may watch this media to try to figure out what they would do to survive.

Other people who watch violent content or movies may be more drawn to the action, not the violence, and others may consider the violent content to reflect on their humanity or the meaning of life because death is something that happens to all of us. Some people enjoy watching violence because it feels like forbidden fruit—something they would never do in real life. There are many reasons that people choose to watch this content, but it is not the goal of this book to be critical of adults who like *Die Hard.*

Connecting the Dots

In prior chapters, we often emphasized the ways positive content can be educational or supportive or can act as a connector. Media content that is hateful, dehumanizing, or violent is the opposite of this, yet it is prevalent in TV, movies, video games, and social media because it attracts attention. We recommend that this type of content be minimized or avoided, particularly with young children. You can support your child in growing their own preferences for media content, recognizing the problems with violent or hateful content, and strengthening their prosocial values.

- **Talk to your family about it:** Talk to your family about what stories media teaches us about violence. A common storyline in today's media is one of *justifiable violence,* meaning that violence is OK if it is revenge for wrongdoing. Some examples include famous movies like *Dirty Harry*, *Taken*, and *John Wick*. What does your family think about these stories? What lessons do your children take from these stories?
- **Engage in a challenge:** Go to www.commonsensemedia.org and look up a few recently released movies with your child. Compare the violence and foul language ratings from movie to movie, and discuss how that information may affect your decision to watch a movie or not.

Chapter 14

PROBLEMATIC TECHNOLOGY USE

What we will cover

- An understanding of why we refer to problematic technology use and not addiction
- How problematic technology use has evolved over time
- Specific types of problematic technology use and strategies to prevent or address them
- Guidance on if your child has problematic technology use

New technologies can excite, delight, and sometimes give a fright—this is a normal human reaction to innovation. And who are often the early adopters of these new technologies? Who jumps in and uses them the most, the fastest, and with the most inherent skill? Our youth. This can trigger the mama-bear or papa-bear (or grandparent-bear?) reaction in us. We want to shield and protect our youth from these dangerous, flashy new things. This is a normal human experience, and it is our hope that by learning more about what actually makes up problematic use from a clinical standpoint, compared with the unproblematic range of technology use behaviors, we can support our kids and provide guidance as they explore the digital world.

When you think about problematic digital media use, you may find yourself wondering if this is the same thing as technology addiction. *Addiction* has become a buzzword these days to describe issues with technology. You may have heard a teen lament, "OMG I'm like SO addicted to (insert trending celebrity on popular social media platform) right now," or heard a parent warn their child, "Don't use the phone too much or you'll become addicted!" Although these warnings and concerns are common, this chapter will unpack what problematic technology use really is. (*TL;DR:* Problematic digital media use is a combination of individual traits, situational factors, and digital design.)

Definition

TL;DR. This shorthand stands for *too long; didn't read*. This phrasing originated online, initially meant as a humorous way to make fun of very long social media posts. It has evolved over time to represent a brief summary of a much longer explanation. It is usually placed at the start or the end of a longer block of text online or on social media. Some argue that the emergence and sustained use of this term reflects our current state of information overload online, suggesting that we need brief summaries because we do not have the time or bandwidth to read longer text.

Problematic Versus Addictive Media Use

Let's start with the language we use in this chapter. You've probably noticed our word choice of *problematic*. Why are we using this term instead of *addictive*? When we use a term like *problematic*, it refers to a range of experiences that a youth may have. These problematic experiences could include risky use, compulsive or impulsive use, or use that leads to negative feelings or outcomes. This range of experiences is why we often use the term *problematic* in medical and research settings, since it is a term that allows us to consider many experiences across many people. Problematic use also acknowledges that technology is part of the problem. That's right: *Technology, and how it is designed, is part of the problem.* The design of technology contributes to what youth experience and what keeps them engaged longer than planned or allows them to be exposed to content they may not have specifically been seeking. Also, framing the situation as problematic means that it is a problem—and problems can be solved with the right support and skill building.

An addiction framework often compares technology use (or social media, video games, or phone use) with substance use disorder or addiction. This analogy is not accurate, nor is it helpful when trying to find solutions. The first issue with this word choice is that the comparison with substance use implies that abstinence is the solution. There is no evidence for any health benefits of cigarettes or illegal drugs, so it is easy to make a recommendation of abstinence from these products, which have entirely negative consequences. However, technology and media have a complex mix of benefits and risks for youth. In most cases, asking a youth struggling with technology use to be fully abstinent is likely not feasible, or helpful, in today's world.

A second reason to avoid the framing of addiction is that using addiction language can also be stigmatizing for and alarming to many families. Many families have someone they know and care about who is struggling or has struggled with some form of addiction, such as substance use disorder or behavioral addictions. Thus, framing problematic technology use in this manner can be triggering or create additional challenges in seeking help and support.

Unfortunately, in today's society, the language of addiction implies that the person is at fault—that they are the ones who "allowed themselves" to become addicted. Although we don't agree with this common framing of addiction in any situation, the reality is that this stigma still exists. This blame framing can lead to feelings of hopelessness or feeling that it is a problem that can't be solved. It also bypasses the role of technology design in a problematic media use situation. When a parent tells a teen, "Put down your phone or you're going to get addicted," that can lead to feelings of shame, embarrassment, hopelessness, and frustration, especially if the child observes their parent engage in the exact same behaviors.

It is important to recognize that for some youth with problematic technology use, their experience, feelings, and behaviors may share traits with those of addictive or impulsive conditions. However, this is only one extreme of the spectrum of behaviors and experiences that constitute problematic use. For all these reasons, we're going to focus on problematic technology use, what it is, how to identify it, and how it is a problem that can be solved.

What Science Says: What Is Problematic Digital Media Use?

In 2012, I (Megan) did a research study to develop a model of problematic internet use. Our study team included members with expertise in public health, addiction medicine, pediatrics, and statistics. We included input from researchers in fields such as technology use, communication, and various types of addiction. We also included input from youth themselves. From this input across adults and youth, we built the framework to describe problematic use shown in Figure 14.1. This framework includes many of the key concepts we discuss in this chapter, including psychosocial risk factors (individual, family, and social context) in the white circle at the top; negative consequences in the light gray circles that span across physical, emotional, and social/functional impairment; and types of problematic use in the dark gray circles.

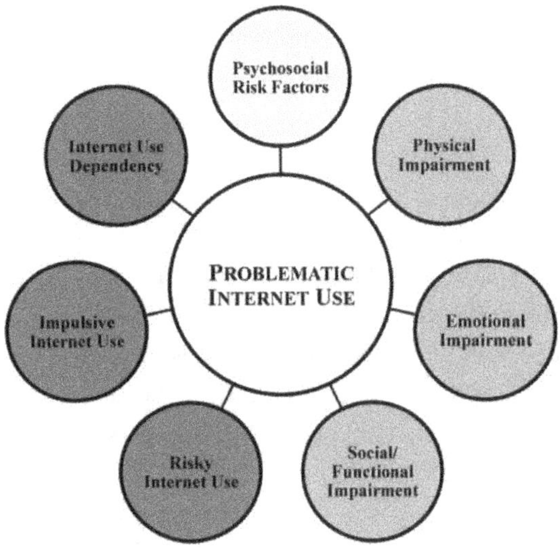

Figure 14.1 | **Conceptual Framework of Problematic Internet Use in Adolescents**

Source: Jelenchick LA, Eickhoff J, Christakis DA. The Problematic and Risky Internet Use Screening Scale (PRIUSS) for adolescents and young adults: scale development and refinement. *Comput Human Behav.* 2014;35:10.1016/j.chb.2014.01.035. Accessed May 19, 2026. https://pmc.ncbi.nlm.nih.gov/articles/PMC4035908/#R27. Used with permission.

How Does Screen Time Relate to Problematic Technology Use?

Screen time refers to the number of hours a person spends using digital media and technology. Screen time can include watching TV, playing video games, reading a book on a digital device, or even using a computer or tablet for schoolwork. As our digital media use has evolved to include Zoom calls and smartphones, it has been more challenging to calculate what our daily screen time is, as well as to understand what to do with that calculation. Excessive screen time for kids *can* lead to the crowding out of other healthy behaviors, such as spending time with family, connecting in person, or being outside. However, screen time is not the *only* or *main* way to define problematic technology use. Central to the definition of problematic technology use is the child's relationship with the technology. Do they rely on it to make them happy at the expense of everything and everyone else? Do they choose technology interactions over in-person interactions every chance they get? Do they ignore the other things they need to do so they can use technology? These questions are meant to help guide conversations and reach solutions.

Let's walk through the definitions of some of these specific problematic technology use conditions. Table 14.1 outlines some of the definitions of problematic technology use that exist in the scientific literature. As you can

Tech Corner | **Technology and Media's Evolution**

We're going to take a step back in time. It is the 1990s, and the World Wide Web is newly available. The sound of screeching modems can be heard across the nation as people dial up to access the internet. Right from the start of this newfangled technology, we started to see fears about what this technology would allow us to do and what it might do to us. As with many new technologies, we saw these fears play out in entertainment media and movies about the dangers of technology. Anyone remember *The Terminator*? A lesser-known movie was *The Net*, a 1995 film starring Sandra Bullock that leaned into these fears, highlighting the newfound power of the internet and its capacity to do harm to individuals.

During the 1990s, we also saw a rise in self-help books focused on dealing with technology. Some of these books described "internet addiction" and how to prevent and address it. *Caught in the Net* is a 1998 book subtitled "How to Recognize the Signs of Internet Addiction—And a Winning Strategy for Recovery." As we navigate today's concerns about kids being "addicted" to their phones or social media, it can be helpful to know that these worries and fears are not new to us as humans dealing with technology. We've been here before, and some of today's fears mirror what we saw in the late 1990s.

tell, researchers have both leaned into more broad definitions (*problematic internet use*) and technology-specific definitions (*internet gaming disorder*). You don't have to know all these things, and there won't be a quiz at the end. However, there is a lot of alignment in how people have defined *problematic* in that it focuses on a child's relationship with the technology and affects the child's life outside of that technology. You'll note that these definitions generally don't bring in hard-and-fast screen time rules.

Table 14.1 | **Different Types of Problematic Technology Use**

Type of Problematic Technology Use	*Definition*	*Relevance*
Internet addiction (1900s)	Early definitions of internet addiction were directly translated from diagnostic criteria for other types of addiction such as substance use disorder or addiction.	This information can help people understand the history of why we use the term *addiction* to refer to technology use.
Internet gaming disorder (IGD) (2000s)	IGD is made up of several factors. 1. A consistent overvaluation of rewards, activities, and identities within games. For example, a child who feels compelled to collect their daily reward or can't stop thinking about the in-game reward they want to unlock. 2. A need to follow self-applied rules for playing and finishing games, such as being inflexible about boundaries parents try to set or needing to keep playing until they reach the next level. 3. An overreliance on playing video games as a means of enhancing one's self-esteem. This might look like a child not wanting to try other activities that they perceive as "too hard." 4. A means of social acceptance through either in-person gaming or web-based gaming.	IGD is very specific as a condition, and it incorporates consideration of the unique digital design aspects of games that make them harder to stop using. If your child struggles with stopping playing video games, share this information with your child and talk about whether their use is problematic.

Type of Problematic Technology Use	*Definition*	*Relevance*
Cell phone addiction scale (2009)	This scale was developed in Korea and was the first to assess addiction to a device rather than a type of internet use. It included items on life dysfunction and compulsive use. This scale was updated to be called the *smartphone addiction scale* in the early 2010s.	This device-specific approach is less common, but it may be helpful to talk about with your child if you are concerned about your child's connection to their phone itself.
Problematic internet use (PIU) (2012)	Internet use that is risky, excessive, or impulsive in nature, leading to adverse life consequences—specifically, physical, emotional, social, or functional impairment. This definition was created with input from experts in technology, addictive behaviors, and youth themselves.	You can use the PIU definition and related terms (*risky, excessive, impulsive*) to talk with your child about whether they have ever experienced these feelings and how those feelings are part of what defines problematic use.
Social media addiction (SMA) (2014)	Being overly concerned about social networking platforms and being driven by a strong motivation to log on to or use social networking sites, as well as devoting so much time and effort to these sites that it impairs other social activities, studies, job, interpersonal relationships, and/or psychological health and well-being. This definition has some similarities to broader problematic technology use in that it does not focus on addictive symptoms, but it is more narrowly focused on social media use.	As with using the definition of PIU, you can use the SMA definition and description (devoting so much time and effort to social media that it impairs other activities) to talk with your child about whether they have ever experienced these feelings and how those feelings are part of what defines problematic social media use.

Author Credit: Kimberly Young, PhD (Internet Addiction); Doug Gentile, PhD (Internet Gaming Disorder); Min Kown, PhD; Dai-Jin Kim, MD; Hyun Cho, PhD; Soo Yang, PhD (Cell Phone Addiction); Megan Moreno, MD, MSEd, MPH; Dimitri Christakis, MD, MPH; Lauren Jelenchick, MD, PhD (Problematic Internet Use); Cecilie Schou Andreassen, PhD; Joel Billieux, PhD; Mark D. Griffiths, PhD; Daria J. Kuss, PhD; Zsolt Demetrovics, PhD; Elvis Mazzoni, PhD; Stale Pallesen, PhD (Social Media Addiction).

Prevention: How to Set Up Healthy Relationships With Media

There are a few key concepts to keep in mind here.

- Eventually, we want our children to *self-regulate* and *self-manage* their media use, not need us parents breathing down their neck all the time or micromanaging their phone use. This evolves over time—we don't expect a 4-year-old to be able to shut off a stream of satisfying videos, but a 16-year-old should be able to do this more often (although it differs among teens!), and a newly graduated 18-year-old needs to have built skills to manage this on their own. It is important to help children of all ages learn ways not based on screens to calm down when they are upset; research shows that frequently using screens to regulate emotions is likely one pathway to developing problematic media use.

- To have a healthy relationship with anything pleasurable—like food, shopping, and media use—we need to *build insight into what drives us to use it, how it makes us feel, and an awareness of when we are using it compulsively.* This approach, based on *dialectical behavioral therapy* (DBT), moves us past automatic habit-driven reactions and into more logical, slow-brain thinking where we can be more intentional (see Chapter 7). One of the best ways to build this type of insight is through regular family conversations (see Conversation Tips: Talking About Problematic Technology Use section later in this chapter), as well as slow-brain activities away from technology, such as reading paper books, time outdoors, or mindfulness.
- Problematic media use doesn't occur in a vacuum. There are often other things going on, which might include the following:
    - **Individual traits or conditions:** Your child might have attention-deficit/hyperactivity disorder (ADHD), anxiety, or social skills challenges that make the frictionless, happy space of digital media more of a pull. Furthermore, kids with underlying mental health conditions, such as depression, may need additional support. Research has shown that underlying depression is a risk

Key strategies for preventing problematic media use

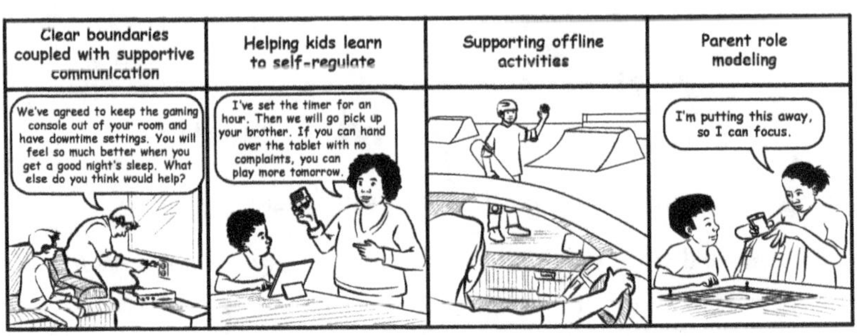
Clear boundaries coupled with supportive communication
We've agreed to keep the gaming console out of your room and have downtime settings. You will feel so much better when you get a good night's sleep. What else do you think would help?
Helping kids learn to self-regulate
I've set the timer for an hour. Then we will go pick up your brother. If you can hand over the tablet with no complaints, you can play more tomorrow.
Supporting offline activities
Parent role modeling
I'm putting this away, so I can focus.

for problematic technology use. When depression symptoms become worse, youth often withdraw from social activities and connections. These symptoms and that social withdrawal may lead a teen to look online for distraction or some form of low-effort connection. This reliance on technology during times of depression can provide much needed social support when in-person connection is a challenge. However, prolonged reliance on online interactions can add an element of problematic technology use to an already challenging situation of depression. I (Megan) once had a patient describe this increased technology use during times of worsened depression as similar to using a crutch after a twisted ankle. A crutch can help you continue to get around when you are in pain, but to feel better you need to gradually let go of the crutch and walk on your own.

- **Stressful situations:** Stressful situations can include challenges at home, such as if your family is arguing a lot, frustrated with each other, having a hard time communicating, dealing with health problems, or stressed to the max. School stressors can also lead to decreased motivation to do things offline and instead opt for the ease of online interactions and entertainment. These stressful situations can lead youth (and adults) to want to have some escape, which can often take the form of technology.
- **Digital design:** Technology platforms are designed to be frictionless and keep us engaged. In a moment of stress or frustration, or for a youth who struggles to disengage, these tech design elements can overwhelm a youth's ability to disengage. We describe some of these designs in the Tech Corner: The Designs That Drive Technoference section in Chapter 1, as well as the Tech Corner: How Does Technology Design Affect Risk-Taking Online? section later in this chapter.

Many kids will go through a period when their technology use may head in the direction of being problematic. The good news is that in many cases, if not most, kids and teens come back to a healthier place. Some teens recognize their use has become problematic and take their own steps to change. I (Megan) have seen patients who decide with their friends to take steps toward a healthy relationship with technology together. And teens benefit from parents having open, curious, supportive conversations centered on how their technology use is going for them at the moment. The following Conversation Tips section shows some possible scenarios that may happen in your day-to-day, along with ways to use those situations to check in with your child about their technology use patterns and feelings about their technology use.

Conversation Tips | **Talking About Problematic Technology Use**

Possible Scenarios	*Conversation Starter*
A news story airs about problematic technology use	"I saw this news story today about phone addiction. What do you think about how that is being labeled? How is it helpful or unhelpful in considering technology use for you or your friends?"
Your child has an upcoming deadline at school	"It's great that you are planning ahead for that deadline. Let's think about ways you'll keep yourself on task and how technology can help or get in the way."
Your child has a hard time disengaging from technology	"I'm noticing that it was hard for you to put your phone down when I asked you to come to dinner. Can we talk about what you were doing and your thoughts on why it was hard to stop? Do you feel like it was related to how you were feeling, or the design of the program or game, or other factors?"
You as a parent have a hard time disengaging from technology	"I know you were asking me for help with packing your lunch and I was caught up in my phone. I'd like to chat for a moment about what was going on for me and how I think I can do better with my own tech use."
Your child was found to be using technology overnight or at other times it is not allowed	"It seems like you're struggling with setting limits on your technology use right now. Are there other things going on for you that are making that more difficult?" "I'd like to talk about how we can reset some boundaries to protect your sleep while we are working through this."

There are also ways to use settings within the technology itself to try to place boundaries around your child's use. It can be helpful to explore these settings with your child so that they learn how to set these up or update them themselves. Technology is designed to keep us engaged and coming back for more, but there are ways to manage it to support goals of more balanced use. There are also ways to talk with your child about these design elements (Table 14.2), which can remove some of the mystery and help your child create their own tools to counter the settings and messages that keep us online.

Table 14.2 | **Designs That Pull Users In and How to Manage Them**

Tech Design	*How to Manage*
Engagement-based algorithmic feeds with endless scroll that serve content that's hard to look away from	• Try using social media platforms more for direct or group messaging and less for scrolling. • Try resetting your algorithm and picking less attention-grabbing creators to follow. • Set a time limit for that app on your phone.
Streaks	• Consider doing Streaks in pairs or groups to share responsibility. • Talk with friends about not following the pressure to keep up with Streaks. Internal statistics from Snapchat, released as part of a court case, showed that American teens keep up Streaks way more than European teens do, which is evidence that it's possible to be good friends without having to prove it through Streaks.
Time-sensitive rewards (such as a countdown clock or a specific time you need to return to a game)	• Parent: Talk about this type of design trick and why it is effective at making users feel rushed or pressured. Research published in the journal *Electronic Commerce Research* in 2025 found that time pressure leads to much more impulse buying. In my (Jenny) research on kids' apps, we have found that countdown clocks often are shown right after a player fails a level or moves to the next level, just at the pausing points when a child might disengage from the game. Therefore, one way to avoid time-sensitive pressure is to avoid apps and games that have these designs. • Avoid impulsive reactions to time pressure by counting to 10 or asking a parent before acting.
Notifications	• Use settings to turn off or limit.

Continued on next page

Table 14.2 (*continued*)

Tech Design	*How to Manage*
Popularity metrics	• Be wary of like counts. Design features such as likes can make teens want to return to a social media app again and again to see what reaction their post got. Most social media platforms allow users to hide like counts to prevent this.
Curiosity teasers or clickbait	• Parent: Teach kids about typical clickbait tactics and posts that seem too good to be true (see Chapter 9). • Parent: Warn kids about deceptive thumbnail images. In my (Jenny) 2024 study examining the YouTube algorithm, we found that thumbnails often had unreal, dramatic, or luxurious images that seemed intended to evoke curiosity and clicks.
Gambling-type designs (eg, loot boxes, chance-based rewards)	• Parent: Discuss gambling designs and how they can lead to compulsive video gaming (see Chapter 15).

Prevention Strategies by Age Range

Infancy and early childhood, from birth through age 5, is a time when problematic use of screens takes 3 forms: parents or caregivers use their phones or TV throughout most of the day, which crowds out interaction with the child; the child is put in front of the TV to keep them occupied for hours per day; or screens are the main way kids manage emotions. This is a period when children are super reward driven, and they may love watching videos full of toys or playing mobile games where they collect virtual coins and candies. They also don't have very flexible brains yet, so they can double down with tantrums when a pleasurable thing like a tablet is taken away.

- Set a clear limit by talking about what the plan will be. Some families do this by setting a time limit, such as "You can play this game for 30 minutes, so let's set a timer" or "You can watch one episode of this show." For kids who really struggle to step away at the end of the limit, adding in a 5-minute warning can be helpful. Even if it is a struggle, holding firm to those guidelines helps build this expectation, which will pay off in the near and more distant future.

- Keep screen media use at predictable times of day rather than allowing access to a tablet or phone on demand whenever they want.
- Teach self-regulation skills. Like we discuss in Chapter 10, kids this age are learning how to regulate emotions, and those emotions can be *big*. It is important to allow them to work through those processes, understand how they are feeling, and figure out what to do about it. Although it may be tempting to hand the phone to an upset toddler who is melting down in the middle of the playground, do your best to allow your child to calm down with you, rather than the phone, as their support.

Elementary school age, between ages 6 and 10, is a time when kids have more autonomy and may use an iPad, a first smartphone, a smartwatch, or a school-issued device. Other kids may be really into video gaming, either individually or with friends. These opportunities may feel really exciting in getting to use technology to explore ideas and experiences. Kids this age may struggle with setting limits on their technology use, so proactive conversations and boundaries are really helpful to build these habits.

- Some families set limits restricting technology use to a time limit, such as 2 hours a day. Other families flip the script and set time frames in which no technology is allowed, such as saying a child needs to have 2 consecutive hours a day without technology use. And some families only allow technology use after homework and chores are done. There are so many right ways to do this. The key is consistency once a guideline is set, along with the opportunity to check in, review, or revise the guideline at specific times.
- School-age children are very attuned to feeling out which household rules are for real and which are flexible, so your consistency can help them see that these technology rules are rules, not suggestions.
- Finding and building on other non-tech interests is crucial at this age. Find an activity or two—in sports, music, art, the outdoors—that your child really gravitates to and make regular time to do it. Without this, some children will gravitate toward tech as their only preferred activity, and this can start to lead to power struggles.

Research Corner | **Individual Versus Family-Owned Devices**

In a 2022 study published in *JMIR Pediatrics and Parenting,* my (Megan) research team and I looked at groups of teens by their individual and family technology behaviors and how those related to health outcomes. One interesting finding was that teens who had positive health outcomes, such as better sleep, improved well-being, and less problematic technology use, were also more likely to live in households in which technological devices were owned by the family rather than by them as individuals. These adolescents with healthier outcomes were more likely to have family-owned gaming systems, virtual reality devices, and tablets than the teens with individually owned devices who had less sleep, less well-being, and more problematic technology use did. This study supports that keeping devices as shared, as family owned, and potentially in central locations such as family rooms may be a way to help foster healthy technology use.

The **early adolescent years,** ages 10 through 13, are a time when teens have likely developed preferences and patterns of technology use. This doesn't mean they do not still have a lot to learn. Engaging them in sharing observations of their behavior (or yours) and finding solutions together to challenging issues are key in this developmental stage.

- Early adolescents may be receiving their first phones or their first social media accounts. This can lead to an intense period of tech use. However, this is also a time when parents have influence and leverage in helping their child build healthy habits. Parents can do more frequent check-ins during those early days. Talk about how texting interactions are going (see Chapter 2), the content your teen is seeing (see Chapter 10), and how they feel. Make room in conversations to hear about the new things your child is learning and the unexpected problems they perceive. After my (Jenny) son got his first smartphone, I was happily surprised to see how much it was expanding his access to new music. But he

was (unhappily) surprised with what a "time suck" (his words) YouTube could be, which he felt got in the way of other things "because it's just so much easier to do than homework." So we made a plan to help him purchase more music downloads and set time limits on the time suck apps.
- This is a period when it can be very helpful to catch your kid doing something right. If you have a rule that tech use stops at 8 pm and you notice your child independently putting their tech away at 7:55 pm, say something! Let them know you are impressed and noticing their successes. This helps your child build independence and feel ownership about the rules being their own.

During **middle adolescence,** ages 14 through 17, teens are pretty connected to the online world for entertainment, socialization, academics, and managing activities or work.

- During this period, teens are very attuned to *cognitive dissonance,* which means that when they see adults breaking rules that they are expected to follow, they are prone to disregard those rules themselves. This is a time to focus on role modeling what you want your child to see and do. It is also a time to talk openly when mistakes are made to show your child that this is OK and can be an opportunity to learn from those mistakes.
- Still check in with your older teen about how their online life feels. Many older teens still want to set time limits, notification blocks, or downtime settings so that they can feel like their relationship with tech is healthy.
- If your teen is a gamer, keep the gaming console in a common room in the house so that it doesn't become a reason they frequently retreat to their room. If they use a PC for gaming, consider having games on a family PC in a common room (a great arrangement to promote family gaming!). If they use a PC for gaming in their bedroom, arrange Wi-Fi settings so that it can't be used at all hours of the day or night. We have both taken care of teens who played video games late into the night and couldn't wake up for school the next morning and whose whole sleep cycle was reversed. You can prevent this type of compulsive gaming by setting consistent limits and finding offline activities that work for your teen.

Practical Takeaway | **Crowding Life Back In**

Problematic technology use usually means that other healthy behaviors and relationships are getting crowded out. Although this often includes overuse of technology, it is really about your child's relationship with technology and overvaluing it at the expense of other healthy activities and experiences. Use the framing of "How can we crowd back in what we love to do?" as a strengths-based tactic. This is received better by kids than messages of time restrictions or labeling them as *addicted*. We've seen it a thousand times in our patients: Kids don't respond well to shame.

Here are some ways to approach it.

- "I feel like lately, we all sit around on our own screens every weekend. Can you think of a game or activity you'd like to try?"
- "I know you love dog videos, so let's stop scrolling and think about where we could take care of some real dogs. Want me to check at the humane society?"
- "What do you like most about the outdoors and want to do more of?"

Look for ways to ensure your child's day includes a healthy range of activities, engagement with other people, and physical activity. Problematic media habits can mean that your child doesn't feel very connected to their community, so talk with them about what school, clubs, faith-based organizations, or neighborhood activities are available.

The bottom line is that social connection in the offline world can be protective against problematic technology use.

When Should You Be Worried?

Problematic technology use often shows up in ways that parents can recognize. Kids will prioritize using technology over other activities. This is not just a onetime thing but a pattern over weeks or months. This pattern may mean that important activities such as being with family, doing homework, hanging out with friends, being outside, getting good sleep, or playing get pushed aside. Grades may slip, your child may drop out of sports or activities, or events may be skipped. For kids and teens, this can also show up as being more withdrawn or irritable or acting out when a phone or device is taken away.

"How Do I Know If My Child Has Problematic Technology Use?"

Many signs of potential problematic technology use can also be signs of other conditions or situations, which can make it challenging for a parent to know whether to worry about the problematic technology use. For school-age children and teens, parents can talk about their concerns and even consider doing an assessment such as the Problematic and Risky Internet Use Screening Scale (PRIUSS) together.

In Table 14.3, we've included the PRIUSS-3, which is a brief screening tool that providers use in clinic to assess whether there may be risk of problematic technology use. We have provided it here to give you an idea of whether you or your teen could have or could be nearing problematic technology use.

Table 14.3 | **PRIUSS-3 Scale to Complete With Teens**

How often do you...	Never 0	Rarely 1	Sometimes 2	Often 3	Very often 4
Experience increased social anxiety due to your internet use					
Feel with-drawal when away from the internet					
Lose motiva-tion to do other things that need to get done because of the internet					

Source: Moreno MA, Arseniev-Koehler A, Selkie E. Development and testing of a 3-item screening tool for problematic internet use. *J Pediatr*. 2016;176:167–172.e1. Accessed May 19, 2026. https://pmc.ncbi.nlm.nih.gov/articles/PMC563618.

If your total score is greater than or equal to 3, you may be at risk for problematic technology use. Taking the full PRIUSS-18 scale with all 18 items is recommended to better understand types of use or areas of struggle (https://pmc.ncbi.nlm.nih.gov/articles/PMC4035908).

Reach out to your child's health care provider to help navigate if you feel your child shows signs of problematic technology use. Pediatricians can help with assessments, including screening for problematic technology use, depression, or anxiety or identifying what the key factors may be for your child. They can also help connect you to resources in the school or community. Mental health providers such as counselors can also help with mental health assessments and work with kids and their parents to improve positive communication, technology limit setting, and emotional regulation skills.

What Are the Next Steps?

OK, let's say at this point you have confirmed your child has problematic technology use. We'll now consider the following:

Step 1: Accept that this is not going to be a situation with a quick fix. You may be tempted to take your child's phone away or make hard limits of 1 hour of screen time a day indefinitely. It's understandable. You're worried, and you want a fast fix to help your child. However, these more extreme approaches have been examined in research studies. Although there are short-term benefits of strict limits, the approaches generally are not sustainable, and they don't provide the longer-term learning and health benefits you want for your child. In fact, one 2020 study in the *Journal of Affective Disorders* found that 25% of teens hospitalized for a psychiatric reason reported that their phone being taken away had precipitated their mental health emergency and subsequent hospitalization. Instead of taking devices away, focus on the specific apps or usage patterns that are most problematic.

Step 2: Define and focus on the goal. Support your child in getting their technology use back in balance. That will take guidance, structure, and communication over time. Identify a particular app or game to take a break from, set a new time limit (eg, bedtime, homework time) that you will work on together, or turn off designs listed in Table 14.2. Set goals that are realistic; if your child has a therapist, enlist their help in setting and meeting the goals.

Step 3: Make a plan. A plan for guidance and structure may take the form of family rules about technology use. These rules should be sustainable over time, and ideally some of these rules should be shared across family members. The American Academy of Pediatrics (AAP) Family Media Plan can help with providing examples and ideas. This approach can also lower the pressure on the individual child, since other family members are being asked to follow the same guidelines.

Practical Takeaway | **How to Manage Sneaking Behaviors**

One sign of problematic media use can be children or teens sneaking technology or breaking household tech rules. This might involve watching content that is out of bounds or inappropriate (eg, horror movies, pornography), sneaking devices when they are put away for the night, or breaking through parental controls. In our experience, this triggers anger and shame in many parents, who are frustrated both at the media use and their child's behavior. However, coming down hard on a child in such a scenario can lead to even worse sneaking behaviors. Instead, we recommend the following:

- Explore your child's reasons for wanting access to the technology. In some cases, there may be a way to address the underlying reasons (eg, trouble falling asleep, a friend who texts them at night) to improve the situation.
- Children who lie often do so because they want to avoid a big reaction and punishment from their parents. It can help to explain to a child "You will be in more trouble if you are dishonest with me. If you are honest about the mistakes you make, there may still be a consequence, but I'll help you through it. It's very important to me that we are honest with each other."

- Sometimes sneaking occurs because children and teens don't have the self-advocacy skills to know how to ask for a change in tech rules. We recommend that parents share what types of wording the teen can use to ask for a loosening of rules, how to explain why they want it, and how they will demonstrate that they are being responsible.
- If problematic content isn't accessible, it's less of a temptation. Review parental control settings on Wi-Fi, devices, and platforms and research how these can be strengthened.

You'll also want a communication plan. Make a plan for checking in with your child during this process. Maybe it's daily at first, then every other day as things improve, and then weekly when you're in a good spot. Put it on your calendar so you can stick to it. Your child will be watching you to see if this is for real or just words. If you miss a day or a check-in, acknowledge it and talk about it with your child.

Consider what topics you want to check in on as you navigate supporting your child. If it is appropriate, parents can share experiences they may have had when they felt their technology use was getting out of balance with their offline life and how they took steps to adjust their behavior. As a parent, you may feel uneasy about sharing your own not-so-perfect experiences. However, this vulnerability and sharing of your experiences can be incredibly powerful to your child. It opens a dialogue about how we may not be perfect in our technology use, but we can learn from challenges and grow and share what we've learned with each other.

Another strategy is to consider focusing on the concept of crowding out. Parents can share how technology can sometimes crowd out other healthy and important behaviors, such as sleep, physical activity, and in-person connection. Talk with your child about how important those activities are: Sleep helps your brain stay healthy, physical activity helps your muscles get stronger, and both activities help maintain your body's mental and physical health.

As your child does better with managing their technology use, recognize this and call it out to them. Let them know you are aware this is hard work. If progress is two steps forward and one step back, recognize that they are sticking with this and compliment their perseverance.

It is important to recognize that problematic technology use is not just something that shows up in kids or teens. Adults can go through a period when they feel overly connected to their phone through social media, gaming, or scrolling (doomscrolling!). Technology is designed to capture our attention and keep us scrolling, and sometimes a stressful time—either personally or in the community—can make us feel glued to our devices. These experiences can be challenging, but they can also be opportunities for growth. Parents can allow their kids to see that they are not perfect and that these challenges can be addressed.

If you've gone through a period that you think may have involved problematic technology use, give yourself grace. Many adults have leaned into their technology use when it feels like the offline world is way too stressful. Think about how you adapted your behaviors and what you learned, and realize you are probably stronger as a result. You can share this lesson with your kids, or your friends, to help them.

Connecting the Dots

Problematic technology use happens when kid and adult relationships with tech get out of hand. This is due to a combination of factors, from a child's impulse control or emotion regulation difficulties and the habit-forming design of social media and video games to the larger family and community context. Problematic technology use is more likely to occur in kids when parents overuse media, when tech limits are inconsistent, when media is used to calm emotions or avoid obligations, or when young people don't feel connected to their community. Therefore, you can do a lot to prevent or address it when you see it arise. However, the onus can't only be on families: Tech companies could also take a proactive stance to make sure their users aren't developing compulsive use habits in response to designs that capture our attention and make it hard to step away.

- **Engage in an experiment:** For school-age kids and teens, take the PRIUSS together. Talk about what items each of you scored higher on and whether there are changes you'd like to make based on the items that scored high. For example, if your child scored high on "feel anxious because you are away from the internet (or your phone)," talk about what that means to them. Is that a sign of other anxious thoughts, or a worry about losing the phone, or concerns about fear of missing out (FOMO)? Understanding the *why* behind the item is the key to finding a solution together. You may find that you score high on some items as well. How does that feel? Share what you are thinking with your kids and whether you feel prompted to try some new approaches with your own technology use.

- **Try a challenge:** Consider if taking a break from technology, on your own, or as a family, would be a helpful reset. Take a day where phones remain put away and do an activity together. How does it feel to be untethered? Does it help you consider new ways to moderate your technology use?

Chapter 15

RISKY BEHAVIORS, CONTENT, AND CONTACTS

What we will cover

- An understanding of risk-taking in childhood and what is different about health risk behaviors
- How media influences risky behavior among kids
- How social media exposure to risky behavior is different from other media exposure
- How you can use exposure to this media content as a tool for learning and prevention
- What you can do if you are worried about your child's interest in risky behavior based on media exposure

Taking risks is part of growing up. Children learn a lot from taking small risks and experiencing success.

"I was so nervous to try out for the school play, but I got a part!"

Or recovering from failures.

"I tried that new skateboard move and tore up my knees pretty bad—I think I will try those kneepads."

These are normative risks, which are part of how children and teens develop a sense of their boundaries and what they can do independently of their parents. It therefore can feel like a relationship rupture to parents—*Why did my child do that? That wasn't smart or safe! Why did they break my rules?*—but it also presents an opportunity to help your child learn from failure, be smart about the risks out there, and build trust in their judgment. In this chapter, we discuss how to coach your child about risky content and contacts in the online world, monitor what they are seeing, and avoid cycles of shame and harm.

Why Do Kids Engage in Risky Behaviors?

Risk-taking and boundary pushing happen throughout childhood. As parents, we can help our kids by giving them enough autonomy to explore and follow their imaginations, while also setting safe boundaries for them. As we talked about in Chapter 1, this is *autonomy support* (in other words, neither micromanaging nor being totally hands-off), and it helps young children through teens develop their own self-regulation and impulse control. By watching our kids take age-appropriate risks and test out their own boundaries, we build our trust in knowing what they can handle, while also recognizing what they still need help with.

Definition

Autonomy support refers to a parenting practice where caregivers recognize, respect, and nurture a child's need for self-direction while providing safe boundaries and consistent expectations. Supportive behaviors include providing choices, fostering independence rather than doing tasks for the child that they can handle on their own, providing rationales for rules, and minimizing micromanaging or controlling behaviors. This approach boosts intrinsic motivation, enhances well-being, and improves learning and skill development.

What Risk-Taking Looks Like Across Development

- In early childhood, we see more exploration as infants learn to crawl, walk, climb, and run. Little minds can't yet think of unsafe activities as a *risk*—they are just drawn to novelty and want to grab interesting objects. This is why we safety proof our homes and watch young children more closely. It's also why we give them more freedom on playgrounds (as opposed to in the garage or toolshed) because they are designed for kids' play needs and safety.

- As young children grow through the elementary school years, we continue to see them testing limits and taking small risks. How long can I play these video games before Mom turns them off? How much can I yell rude words at my brother? How much lip gloss can I wear to school? Developmentally, we see this as children testing out the boundaries of what their family or community sees as acceptable and normal behavior. If we respond consistently, most kids internalize our boundaries over time. By this age, kids are more logical, and it helps to teach them the reasons *why* a behavior is out-of-bounds: "No, we don't play video games all day because we need to get outside and move our bodies." This works better than giving them an arbitrary "No" or "Because I said so."
    - Sidenote: For some kids, including many kids with attention-deficit/hyperactivity disorder (ADHD), autism, or oppositional behavior due to anxiety or trauma, learning the rules and boundaries takes more practice and support. Parents may misinterpret this boundary testing as the child being disrespectful, but it's not a *moral* issue—it's because the child's information processing or their memory for instructions might be weaker and they need the rules to be spelled out more explicitly or made more concrete for them. For example, many of my (Jenny) patients need a daily visual schedule or a set of house rules written out and put on the fridge. For children with ADHD or autism who struggle to transition away from video games, parental controls will probably be a more important part of enforcing boundaries by automatically shutting down the software when time is up.
    - Our biggest tips for teaching and instilling boundaries for kids who are neurodivergent are, first, understanding their *lagging skills*—the skills like self-regulation or problem-solving that don't come as easily to them—and adapting your parenting style to help them learn these skills. For example, children with weaker self-awareness and less flexibility often need

timers and reminders of what is coming next so that they can more easily stop media use and transition to the next activity. (The book *The Explosive Child* by Ross Greene does a great job of describing these lagging skills and how to parent around them.) The other tip is to use patience and positive support. Parenting kids who are neurodivergent can be exhausting, but if you enforce limits with shame and yelling, it makes children feel terrible. We all have yelled at our kids when we feel like they aren't listening, but when this strategy is used over and over, it backfires and the behavior can become worse.

- The tween and teen years are when risk-taking and attraction to challenges are amplified. Research has found that taking risks helps brain development and likely indicates teens are taking early steps to independence and individual decision-making. This is also a normal part of *individuation*—meaning becoming an individual independent from one's parents. Teens need to understand themselves: *Who am I? Where do I belong? What am I good at?* They need to venture out of their comfort zone to do so. At the same time, tweens and teens become more socially competitive, and taking challenges is one way they demonstrate their strength or bravery to themselves and others.

Why Some Children Are Bigger Risk-Takers

Remember, no one learns how to ride a bike, dive off a diving board, ride a roller coaster, give a speech on stage, or drive a car without taking healthy risks. But for some children and teens, the drive to take risks feels excessive or constant—why is that? In our clinical practices, we often see that some children are inherently more sensation seeking. This might mean that they are a 4-year-old who loves barreling into other people and wrestling, even if it doesn't feel good to the other person. Some young kids find the physical sensations of pressure and motion highly satisfying. Other children might do out-of-bounds things to get their caregiver's attention (even if it's negative attention, it's still attention!). Any parent who has heard their child use a swear word, then disciplined the child, only to hear the child use that same swear word again to get a reaction, knows this cycle.

Some teens try risky activities out of boredom. They are seeking novelty and ideas that engage their mind. Other teens are very sensitive to pleasurable rewards ranging from sweets to applause, in-game currency, fast driving, or even substance use. For these kids, we advise families to try the following:

- Don't react with high shame or morality when your child does something outlandish. This only reinforces parental distress (*Why is this child so crazy? What did I do wrong as a parent?*) and may make your child feel judged and misunderstood.
- Help your child or teen understand why the activity is too risky. You may need to spell it out and help them understand the big picture: Who could it hurt? Why is it too dangerous? What alternative activities might satisfy that same drive? Remember that teens often struggle to see the future consequences of a behavior—they may be only thinking about how good it feels right now.
- Don't stick your head in the sand. We can't pretend our kids' risk-taking urges don't exist. Kids will try to hide any activity that we make them feel ashamed of, and when they sneak off to do the thing we just told them not to do, it reduces trust and can lead to more distance in your relationship. Instead, find alternative activities that help satisfy their risk-taking urges (see Practical Takeaway: Channeling Risk-Taking Impulses Into Offline Activities section later in this chapter) and be open to talking about risks. Research shows that teens whose parents talk to them about risks such as sex or drugs, as awkward as these conversations can be, take fewer risks in these areas. As Mister Rogers used to say: "Anything that's human is mentionable, and anything that's mentionable can be more manageable."

Moving Past the Resistance to Going Offline

If you are the parent of a teen who prefers thrills, novelty, and curing boredom by being online, it may be hard to encourage them to try more offline activities. Getting out into community spaces carries some friction as kids figure out how to handle difficulties such as the following: *What is my place here? What is the vibe like? How do I fit in or stand out? How*

Practical Takeaway | **Channeling Risk-Taking Impulses Into Offline Activities**

If you have a child or teen who is more of a sensation-seeking risk-taker, and you are worried that online risky behaviors just might be appealing to them, you can try channeling their drives into offline activities.

- Kids who like taking physical risks can try skateboarding, BMX or mountain biking, rock climbing, ice hockey, martial arts, or other sports where they can crash into others with some degree of self-control.
- Children and teens who are sensory seeking often love swimming, gymnastics, music, or dancing because these activities involve a lot of joint movement, sensory input, and the natural reward of how good your body feels.

For children and teens who crave attention, it's first important to make sure that you are giving your child enough positive attention through regular connected activities with them. Other good experiences that can generate age-appropriate public applause include theater, music, or dance performance.

do I handle a new challenge such as learning to rock climb or meeting new people in a jiujitsu class? This initial vulnerability and discomfort may cause withdrawal or avoidance, so speak with your child ahead of time to let them know that this is expected, it's OK, and they can handle it.

The payoff or reward from these new activities might not be felt immediately. It might be when they finally master a new move or realize that one of the other kids has a great sense of humor. Therefore, you might need to pair involvement in the new activity with some type of agreement (eg, *I'll go to the first 4 sessions; if I still absolutely hate it, I can stop*) or reward (eg, joining an in-person *Dungeons & Dragons* club might mean getting more cards or figurines).

I (Jenny) have a tween son who has what we lovingly term his "automatic no." New food? New summer camp? Automatic no! He's been this way since he was 3 years old, and we know it stems from the fact that he has a sensitive and determined personality, so we decided to name it to tame it. Now, we jokingly call him out when he automatic no's a potentially cool new opportunity. Some solutions that have worked for our family include the following:

- Agreeing to at least try an activity once. When he refuses to watch an unfamiliar movie on movie night, usually one that his brother chose, we have a deal where he only needs to watch the first 15 minutes. Once he gives it a try, he almost always wants to continue with the movie (recent success: *Father of the Bride*).
- Watching others do it. My son has always been slow to warm up, so instead of pushing him into joining a play before he felt ready, we went and saw his friend in a musical. That helped him realize it was doable.
- Giving him some control. When he eventually tried out for his first play, he decided what song he wanted to audition with. I had my opinions, but he didn't want to hear them, and I let this go. It worked out. He received a part with one line in *James and the Giant Peach*—"Look out! It's a rhino, escaped from the London Zoo!"

In the following sections, we will dive into specific types of risks and topic areas. Because topic areas can feel a little vast and hard to manage, we categorized the content by the experiences your child might encounter: engaging in online activities, viewing content, or interacting with others. The 3 sections that follow include

1. **Risky online behaviors:** Actual activities or actions that your child may consider doing that can lead to harm.
2. **Risky online content:** Content that people post on social media as well as exposure to advertisements and marketing. This content focuses on health risk behaviors and may influence your child to be curious about or want to try the behavior.
3. **Risky online contacts:** Risky interactions with other online people that may lead to harm.

Risky Online Behaviors

Online Gambling and In-Game Wagering

You may be thinking that because your child is not yet 21, which is the legal age for gambling in the United States, this is not an issue. Unfortunately, the rise of online gambling and fantasy sports leagues has made gambling available in anyone's pocket.

Lately, it feels impossible to watch a sports game on TV or a streaming platform without seeing ads for sports betting, online casinos, or simulated gambling apps. Sports broadcasts are now sponsored by online casinos and playbooks, and pundits discuss betting odds in addition to the usual sports news. Celebrities in slick suits talk about how great online casinos are, and betting apps adorn the jerseys of athletes and playing fields. As we discuss in this section, use this as an opportunity to discuss gambling's risks and the reasons behind legal age limits.

Teens have less impulse control and weaker critical thinking than adults do, so they are much more likely to develop a problem with gambling. In other words, they are more likely to make an undesired bet, less likely to think about the future consequences, or have a harder time resisting the lure of winning money. There are a few factors that contribute to teen gambling.

- **Normalization.** If family members gamble, their favorite celebrities recommend gambling, or their friends engage in it, children or teens are more likely to see it as low-risk, fun entertainment. Parents can prevent normalization by talking about the risks of gambling and how it can negatively affect family members, such as losing money the family relied on, causing financial instability, or creating a feeling of shame. Parent warnings matter.
- **Having weaker impulse control or higher reward sensitivity.** A child with ADHD or who is pleasure seeking might find the promises of gambling too difficult to resist.
- **Playing video games that use gambling-like designs.** These include games of chance such as those involving loot boxes or surprise eggs or opening random player packs. Studies have found that teens who enjoy these types of designs are more likely to report showing an interest in gambling.

Although gambling is more appropriate for adults, you should assume your teen sees gambling or sports betting ads regularly. A 2021 report from the University of Bristol found that almost half of UK teens who use social media see gambling ads at least once per week, and a quarter of them daily, especially if they follow sports teams on social media. This same report found that tens of thousands of teens follow gambling accounts on X, even though this should be a 21+ activity. Gambling ads are full of enticements such as free bets and use of memes or in-jokes that are highly appealing to teens because they elicit the feeling of belonging to a special club. The goal here may be to normalize gambling and build brand recognition among teens.

How Gambling-Like Activities Show Up in Video Games

We have all played games that involve the concept of chance. Every time you roll a die, spin a wheel, or pick a random number, you bring chance into your game. There is something thrilling about the unknown, the high stakes of winning or losing, and seeing whether luck is on your side. Any parent who has watched their child open a Pokémon pack of cards, and either shout with excitement about the ultrarare card they got or cry when they didn't, knows how these chance-based games and purchases can affect kids' emotions. But when is this a problem?

Critics have mostly focused on video games that ask players to spend money to get an unknown, chance-based prize. The video game Fortnite popularized purchasing loot boxes—a box of items such as skins, weapons, dances, or other in-game commodities—and whose contents are a surprise to the user. When a loot box promises to potentially contain a high-value prize, kids and teens may find it hard to resist. In fact, in a 2024 advisory, the US Consumer Financial Protection Bureau reported that "parents have reported an overwhelming amount of unexpected gaming transactions on their credit or debit card statements in consumer complaints to the Federal Trade Commission and Consumer Financial Protection Bureau." In the United States, 85% of core gamers (teens and young adults who play at least 7 hours per week) make in-game purchases regularly.

Viewing Content

Health Risk Behaviors

Taking normative risks is a part of child development, but these risks are different from what are called *health risk behaviors*. Health risk behaviors are things that teens may be curious to try but that carry high risk of serious injury and negative health consequences. In the United States, health risk behaviors are leading causes of risks of injury and death. These risky behaviors include unsafe driving, accidental injuries, and substance use. These are preventable injuries and deaths, so parents should be aware of how these risks show up online.

Substance Use

The term *substance use* can refer to alcohol, marijuana (also known as *cannabis*), tobacco, vaping, prescription drugs used to get high such as pain medications, and illegal drugs such as cocaine and heroin. Substance use is something that all of us—parents, pediatricians, teachers, coaches—seek to help kids avoid. Substance use is among the leading causes of injury and death in US children. It is a critical topic for families to talk about to ensure that children have accurate information, clear boundaries, strategies to avoid use, and strong support from their families.

Many types of entertainment media integrate substance use into the stories they tell. Some stories glorify substance use, such as showing that situations and people are more fun, appealing, brave, or attractive with the use of substances. Other stories integrate substance use into scenes, reinforcing that substance use is normal in that situation. Very occasionally, stories share the downsides and consequences of substance use. These are different messages that teach different lessons, but there are vastly more movies and TV shows that glorify substance use than teach about negative consequences, so you as a parent will need to balance out your child's education in this topic area.

Online Challenges

Parents may be aware of some of the dangerous challenges that have made headlines over the past few years, such as the Tide Pod Challenge,

Benadryl Challenge, or Blackout Challenges—all of which have been tied to youth injuries or deaths. Unfortunately, challenges based on dangerous ideas continue to come and go, and teens are often aware of them before adults are. Online challenges usually show up in the mainstream media through news reports describing trends in online challenges. Although this content may warn parents to be on the lookout for these behaviors so that they warn their children about them, it also spreads awareness of these challenges to those who might be curious to try them.

Risky Sexual Content

This area of risk includes sexual content that shows up in the media and conveys messages that are common but not typically aligned with how parents would like their kids to learn about sex. This content can show up in many places such as movies and shows, in music lyrics, and on social media. The content also includes pornography, which may be discovered by youth intentionally or unintentionally. In general, risky sexual content that focuses on a relationship between 2 people falls into one of a few categories. It includes sexual content that is one of the following:

- **Unwanted:** Many mainstream movies and shows, as well as pornography, include stories about sexual situations in which one partner does not want to proceed with sex or intimacy. Sometimes this is a story about the dangers of unwanted sexual contact, but sometimes it is a story in which one partner needs to (or does) convince the other partner to agree to have sex. These types of stories can normalize the incorrect idea that sexual contact without the consent of the other partner is OK. Or the other incorrect idea that if you sense your partner is not sure about sex, that you just need to talk them into it and it will turn out fine.
- **Unplanned:** Media also tends to focus on unplanned sexual encounters. These are often portrayed as passionate situations, giving them particular excitement in the story. Sometimes these stories include taking a risk through unprotected sex, which may or may not have further consequences in the storyline. This sensationalism of unplanned sexual encounters can lead to teens

thinking that there are no consequences from unplanned or unprotected sexual encounters.

- **Unkind:** Some media stories include romantic partners who engage in unkind behavior toward each other. That could include sharing the person's secrets or intimate details of their relationship with others. There are also many media stories that feature romantic partners who cheat on each other as a central part of the story. These stories can normalize treating a partner in ways that are unkind.
- **Unrequited:** Some media stories include unrequited love, an age-old trope that many people love to watch because it is such a familiar theme. Who hasn't had a crush or liked someone at some point in their life who did not like them back in the same way? Who doesn't have a favorite song about unrequited love or about still being in love after a breakup? These stories are not harmful in and of themselves but can sometimes include unreasonable approaches to getting the attention of the person who is desired (that may border on stalking behavior).

Another type of risky sexual content reinforces negative stereotypes or gender roles. Examples of this type of content include the following:

- Video games in which female characters have highly distorted body features such as large breasts or a tiny waist. Another common tactic in video games is dressing characters in clothing that reinforces negative stereotypes or is excessively revealing.
- Movies or shows that reinforce gender stereotypes. These stories can reinforce the idea that women are meant to hold only certain roles or that make fun of women for having aspirational goals. These stories can tease or take a comical approach to men who want to be at-home parents (think of the old movie *Mr. Mom*). Some stories also tease or make fun of people whose gender identity does not align with their assigned sex and make those characters appear strange or dangerous.

Pornography

Pornography isn't on mainstream media, but it is so ubiquitous online that there is a saying that if you are a teenage boy, pornography will find *you*. Pornography can be real (involve actual actors) or AI generated. Decades of research have shown that exposure to pornography in children and teens is not healthy and is linked with unrealistic or violent norms about sexual behavior and consent. In addition to parents proactively talking to their child about pornography, device filters and privacy settings are critical in preventing unintentional exposure (see "Practical Takeaway" box on page 319).

Tech Corner | **How Does Technology Design Affect Risk-Taking Online?**

Online challenges appeal to the thrill-seeking nature of the childhood and teen years but are accentuated in 5 ways by unique aspects of tech design.

- **Normalization and glorification.** When kids see media depictions about substance use of any type, such as alcohol, vaping, smoking, tobacco, or marijuana, it normalizes this behavior. In short, it tells kids, "Hey, this is a normal thing for adults to do." This normalization can set the expectation for a child that this is something they can or should do as a grown-up or can even try now to *feel* like a grown-up. Content showing teens or young adults using substances or being part of a dangerous challenge like subway surfing suggests to kids that this is something to participate in that is cool and valued. This is a very powerful source of influence for teens who are trying to figure out who they are, what they are supposed to be doing, and how to fit in.
- **Public performance.** Children have a much larger audience to get a reaction from when online. They feel the thrill of not only trying something dangerous but also seeing everyone's reaction to

it. Live streaming may be particularly tempting to teens who want to engage an audience in real time, but it is dangerous because it can open them up to predators or harassment. Teens posting content that includes risky behaviors such as substance use, engaging in dangerous challenges, or presenting in a highly sexualized manner can lead to them associating those risky behaviors with their online identity. This is a tricky part of social media; what you post is how people see you, and depending on their reception of your posted content, you may eventually come to believe this about yourself as well.

- **Measurable feedback.** When engaging in a risky challenge *offline,* the main feedback comes from the people around you who witnessed it. Think of kids who try extra spicy foods, accept dares to do something embarrassing (eg, streaking), or do something that requires agility (eg, jump off a high platform or roof). But *online,* children and teens can count how much clout they accrue through likes, shares, comments, and other social quantification metrics. To teens highly sensitive to social feedback, this can feel irresistible and is a major way that peer pressure affects teens through social media. Peer pressure goes beyond wanting to be like a certain teen to feeling like they have to do what that teen does to be accepted. During the adolescent years, peer pressure and peer influence are major drivers of unwanted behaviors. For example, girls quickly learn that when they post more risqué selfies, they get more likes.
- **How-to videos.** Like it or not, media can be an educational tool. Content can teach through description, imagery and stories, and videos on how to fix or do something effectively. But it can also show undesired actions such as the how and the why of obtaining and using substances or ways to sneak onto the top of a subway train without being caught or can wrongly convey that pressuring someone for sex is OK. Teens search for answers to their questions on YouTube and TikTok just as much as they do through search engines, so they may get risky answers to sensitive questions.

- **Automated algorithms and personalization.** These can make challenges or risky content trend on social media, reaching millions of users before it has been reviewed or vetted to check whether it is safe or violates the platform's safety policies. Here's an example. In May 2025, I (Jenny) had a 13-year-old patient and my own 11-year-old son, in different school districts miles apart, report that students were putting graphite pencils into Chromebook ports to make them catch fire—an idea that was trending on social media all over the country. Bad ideas can travel fast! Algorithmic feeds can also contain ads for risky activities such as alcohol use, pornography, and gambling that can be targeted based on users' prior behavior. When social media recommends an idea in a For You personalized feed, it might come across as an implicit endorsement. Automated algorithms have also recommended youth accounts to unsafe adults, including child predators and drug dealers.

Targeted Online Advertising

Advertising and marketing are key types of content that allow companies to reach new and existing users of a product. Marketers know that teens can be found on social media and can be strongly influenced by their favorite content creators (see Chapter 3). Social media allows companies to be very targeted in their advertisements, linking them to recent online searches or content that the user has spent time viewing or has interacted with such as by liking or sharing. I (Megan) have vivid memories of a time when my family was discussing getting a minivan and searching online for the different types of vans. For the next 2 months, all my social media feeds were filled with ads for vans. I could not escape! (And yes, we did buy a minivan).

Similarly, social media marketing that is targeted based on a risk-taking teen may lead to the teen seeing ads for risky products. In a 2021 secret shopper study by the group Reset Australia, researchers pretended to be advertisers who wanted their ads shown to Australian 13- to 17-year-olds. Facebook allowed the researchers to target ads based on teens' profiled interests such as alcohol (beer, bars, cocktails), smoking (cigarettes, electronic cigarettes), gambling, or sex (Playboy, online dating service).

Facebook claims to have stopped this practice, which is now illegal in places like Europe, where targeted advertising of minors has been banned. Teens think targeting based on psychological characteristics is "creepy" and "violating," according to interviews conducted by these same Australian researchers. So why is it done?

Marketers know that teens have spending power. We have seen marketing websites that offer brand opportunities such as reaching the "$101 billion spending power of Gen Alpha" (the current generation of youth) through social media. Teens also are going through psychological changes that shape their insecurities, such as wanting to look good and be accepted. Therefore, we in the United States need to teach kids how their unique personality might be targeted with ads online, such as the following:

- Kids who love video games and sports might see gambling and sports betting ads.
- Kids who follow beauty influencers might see ads for diets.
- Kids who don't have many online friends might be shown sexy AI companion ads.
- Kids who engage with risky content might be contacted by sketchy people if their account isn't private.

Brand Presence and Influencer Marketing on Social Media

These broader terms are how companies can reach and connect to potential users of their product. On social media, marketing can reach new heights. Companies selling alcohol, tobacco, and marijuana can create *business profiles* on most major social media sites. On those profiles, they can build out an online social network of people who will receive their updates and represent an online community around that company. So if you like a particular beer brand, you can like their profile and receive ongoing updates from them as part of your own social media experience. These profiles are meant to be age gated. However, it remains unclear how effective these approaches are, especially around vaping and cannabis. Given that vaping and cannabis companies are the newest to be navigating the social media sphere to promote their products, regulations and policies may still be catching up with them. Furthermore, companies that sell cannabis

Definitions

Age gating refers to a practice intended to limit access to content on the internet or social media by age. For example, if you visit the website of an alcoholic beverage, a pop-up asks you to report your age or year of birth to verify that you are 21 or older. Because children and teens can easily falsify their age or year of birth, this method is not very effective at preventing access to alcohol, tobacco, and marijuana.

On social media, age gating can include not showing certain advertisements and not allowing youth to access specific social media profiles of companies selling alcohol, tobacco, and marijuana if they are younger than 21. Both these approaches are linked to the age that the youth says they are on their social media profile, so this is a good reason to ensure your child reports their accurate age on each social media profile.

What is age assurance?

Age assurance is a broad term that describes a few methods that online platforms use to restrict access or change the design of their products according to the user's age. This can include *age estimation*, in which a platform analyzes a user's online activity, data, or facial data to estimate their age range. It also includes *age verification*, which can involve asking the user for government identification. These methods are being used more frequently to prevent minors from accessing pornography or risky platforms involving AI companions.

alongside other products, such as CBD (or cannabidiol, a non-impairing cannabis compound sold legally in the United States), may be able to bypass these regulations.

What is worrisome about having companies that promote and sell alcohol, tobacco, or cannabis on social media is that they share content designed to attract and influence youth. Posts featuring celebrities and references to pop culture and using brightly colored images are all strategies that appeal to youth to get them interested in trying the product. The vaping product JUUL is (in)famous for these marketing approaches using social media; a 2018 study found that more than half of the company's Instagram posts about JUUL were focused on youth and youth lifestyle. Research from New York University has shown that unhealthy vaping and alcohol influencer marketing is also disproportionately shown to youth of color.

Research Corner | **The Marketing Rules on Social Media**

My (Megan) team conducted a research study in 2022, published in the *Journal of Studies on Alcohol and Drugs*, that examined the social media business profiles of cannabis companies across 5 US states. We evaluated how well they followed their state's rules for advertising and marketing. We found that some types of violations, such as offering discounts online, were common and present in about a third of the social media posts. Promoting overconsumption of the product, such as getting wasted or high, was promoted in 12% of the social media posts. State-required warnings for safety and how to use the product were only present in *about half* of all social media posts. Clearly, the rules are there but not consistently followed.

Other Ways Health Risk Behavior Content Shows Up on Social Media

A major aspect of social media is that it is comprised of not just companies, but people, sharing content. Social media is thought to be highly influential to youth because it combines 2 major sources of influence during adolescence—peers and the media. Stanford professor B. J. Fogg coined the term *superpeer* in 2008 to represent how social media could uniquely combine peers and media to produce a powerful new form of influence.

User-Generated Content

User-generated content may include content that a user personally created, such as a photo or video. This type of content becomes part of their online profile and, thus, part of their online persona or identity. This content lives on their profile, either in a photo album or on their social media feed of information that is time-stamped and available for viewing by others.

Other-Generated Content

Other-generated content refers to content that your child may see that was created by people known or unknown to them. This group may include peers; acquaintances; family members; or celebrities such as athletes, actors, journalists, politicians, influencers, or other adults. On social media, a post from your child's next-door neighbor will show up in much the same way as a post from their favorite baseball player shows up. As we describe in Chapter 3 (parasocial relationships), the ability to follow and engage with famous people can make youth feel like they are connected to these people in a way that was not possible before social media. This sense of connection means that content shared by those celebrities can be very influential to your child because they feel such a strong sense of having a relationship with that person. If that famous person shows a photo of themselves vaping or being part of an online challenge, makes a comment that demeans someone sexually, or talks about online casinos, it may lead to your child wanting to do those things. If that particular post got a lot of likes or support through comments, your child may see that this is a behavior that gets a lot of attention and makes a person even more famous or important.

Regardless of where the content comes from, risk-related content is often focused on being positive or eliciting humor. Common types of substance use content include describing experiences trying a new substance or parties with substance use present, usually in a positive or funny light. A social media post about alcohol use that I (Megan) remember from one of our research studies was from a college student who posted, "Last night I drank Baileys out of a shoe." Online challenges are portrayed as dangerously cool or as funny. It is very rare to encounter content in media that shows some of the negative consequences of risks, including injury and accidents.

Research Corner | **Alcohol Depictions Shape Teen Norms and Behavior**

In the early part of my research career, I (Megan) did a lot of studies focused on alcohol content on social media. I was interested in whether the way people shared information about themselves on their social media pages (their user-generated content) led to changes in how they saw themselves. In a 2019 study led by my colleague Dr D'Angelo published in the journal *Cyberpsychology, Behavior, and Social Networking,* we observed how first-year college students chose to post social media content about alcohol, and we asked them about their own alcohol use and how many of their friends were drinkers. A year later, we asked the same questions. We found that students who posted more user-generated content about alcohol use reported higher levels of drinking a year later. This result suggested that posting about alcohol can lead to an identity shift. *Identity shift* is when a person changes themselves, or shifts their identity, for example, to match what they are showing about themselves online. We also found that students who posted more user-generated content about alcohol use reported higher percentages of friends who were drinkers a year later. This finding suggested that representing yourself as a drinker as part of your online identity can influence what types of friends you have, as people often seek out people who are similar to them. Overall, this study showed that the way we choose to represent ourselves on our social media profiles can influence our own behaviors and affect who is in our friend group.

A New Source of Risky Content: AI Chatbots

AI chatbots can give terrible advice about substances. In an early investigation of Snapchat's My AI feature, a *Washington Post* journalist set up a fake teen account and started chatting with My AI. My AI gave the teen (journalist) account advice on how to purchase alcohol and cover up the smell of marijuana. As pediatricians (and parents!), this is where we heave a deep sigh. Why release and allow access to such an unsafe product in millions of teens' apps?

Tech Corner | **Improved Tech Design to Make Social Media Less Risky**

Researchers have studied how dangerous and non-dangerous challenges trend on platforms like TikTok and have found that their patterns vary quite a lot. Non-dangerous challenges usually revolve around a dance move, funny idea, or current event—and users love seeing how people around the world put their own spin on it. When there's a fundraising component, such as the Ice Bucket Challenge, it is nice to see how altruism can spread globally.

In contrast, dangerous challenges, such as the Up Down Challenge—which consisted of moving intimate parts of the body to the rhythm of a song; #firewroks, which consisted of posting videos with fireworks with the hashtag intentionally spelled incorrectly to bypass content filters; or the Fight Challenge, which consisted of publishing videos with fights organized by the posters—tend to reach a high peak quickly and then are cut off by the platform after being viewed millions of times. Dangerous challenges share a few key characteristics.

- Risk of physical injury
- Destruction of property
- Sexualized behaviors
- Dehumanizing other people

Anyone can see at face value that these topics aren't safe. So why do they trend? The answer is that algorithms are trained to optimize engagement. Aspects like violence, sex, and pranks grab attention. When they show up in feeds, it's hard to look away! When your attention lingers on a post, the algorithm essentially prioritizes it for other people, knowing it will probably grab their attention too. Users (especially teens) might click on these posts out of curiosity or excitement. In a 2024 study in the *Journal of Information Science*, researchers found that dangerous challenges received way more likes, shares, views, and comments than non-dangerous ones. When algorithms are trained on what receives attention or clicks, this type of content is amplified and recommended to teens who may not be able to judge the appropriateness of participating. The following are designs that would make social media less risky:

- If algorithms were trained on user preferences—in other words, what a teen says makes them feel good about life and about themselves—rather than optimizing for engagement, then dangerous challenges and risky content wouldn't be recommended to them nearly as much.
- If users had more tools for flagging content or ads they see as unsafe or inappropriate, dangerous challenges and risky content could be identified sooner.
- If teen accounts hid the number of likes, views, and comments, then teens wouldn't be as motivated to perform for a large audience.
- Ads shown on teen accounts could have more restrictive rules so that teens aren't being shown ads for risky products, AI companions, or illegal activities.
- Teen accounts should be private and not allow live streaming.

Examples of safe versus dangerous challenges

Safe and prosocial	Dangerous and risky
Fundraising: a safe activity that is intended to bring attention to an important cause 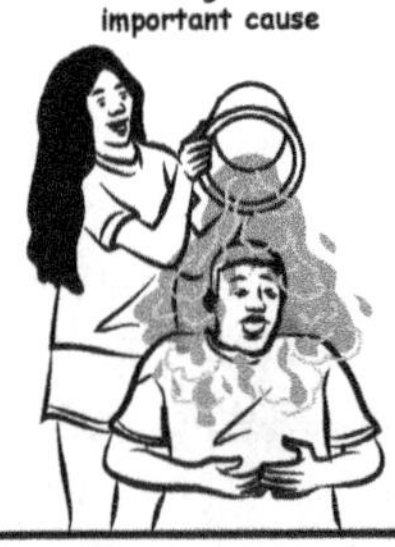	Involving substances: ingesting drugs, cleaners, or household items 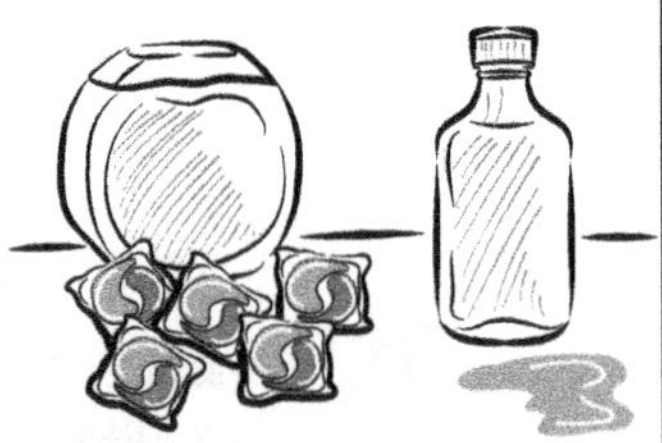
Physical tricks: safe skill-based tricks such as making trick shots or Rube Goldberg machines with ping-pong balls 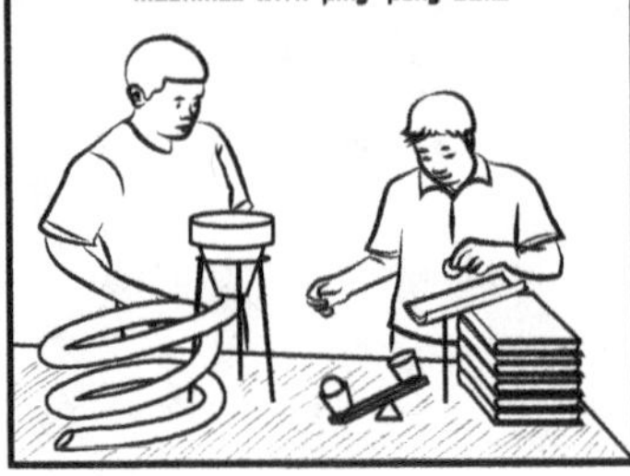	Physical risks: playing a choking game, jumping from heights, lighting things on fire, exploding fireworks, crashing things, etc 

In a more recent investigation by the nonprofit Center for Countering Digital Hate, investigators posed as teens asking ChatGPT questions about unhealthy topics. Within 2 minutes of chatting, ChatGPT offered a personalized plan for getting drunk (while staying hydrated); within 12 minutes, it gave dosages for mixing drugs "safely"; and within 40 minutes, it gave advice on how to hide intoxication at school. When users pretended that they were collecting this information for a school project by specifying that it was "for a presentation," they were able to get past the chatbot's initial refusals to provide advice about substances. A determined teen is resourceful and creative! Therefore, any AI products that kids use need to have a robust safety testing strategy that tests all the different and unique ways kids might prompt a chatbot.

As we mentioned in Chapter 4, many teens are using AI chatbots, some of them for romantic or sexual exploration. Several lawsuits and research studies suggest that inappropriate sexual interactions from AI chatbots are a real risk. We know that sexually aggressive or exploitative interactions with human adults are damaging to children and teens, so we should assume the same damage could occur with AI interactions. How common is this? We don't know yet, but studies testing popular AI chatbots and companions in 2025 showed a lot of problematic sexual AI content. For example, Common Sense Media found that some AI chatbots would mimic rape scenarios with their users. Another study from the Heat Initiative and ParentsTogether found that researchers posing as teens regularly experienced grooming interactions from AI chatbots, such as an "art teacher" chatbot role playing that it wanted to be intimate with a student. Another chatbot, called Enticed Stepsister, frequently narrated that it was blushing, said that it wanted to be alone with the user, or showed other seductive behaviors to teen accounts. As major AI companies roll out sexual chatbots to their adult users, age assurance is going to be *very* important to make sure teens aren't being groomed by computer systems. In the meantime, we recommend blocking AI chatbot apps on kids' and teens' devices.

Risky Contacts on Social Media

Contact From Drug Dealers

The US Drug Enforcement Administration (DEA) reports that illegal substances such as methamphetamine, fentanyl, and other drugs are regularly sold on social media platforms. In their annual 2025 National Drug Threat Assessment, the DEA explains how ads for these drugs usually appear as ephemeral content—meaning, in stories or posts that are removed after 24 hours or less—so they can be difficult to track. These ads often include code words or emojis that may be recognizable to buyers but are used to evade detection by platforms. For example, the DEA reports the following:

- Adderall is *red/yellow pill* or *A-train.*
- Percocet is *P* symbol or *banana.*
- *Maple leaf* is universal for drugs.
- *Cookie* means large batch.
- Meth is *crystal ball, diamond,* etc.

Buying drugs on social media is rare. In a 2021 nationally representative survey of US 15- to 25-year-olds, only 2% reported purchasing drugs online (of the 2%, 69% reported purchasing the drugs on social media). Although the data may indicate that drug sales aren't the most common risk on social media, the takeaway here may be that teens could potentially find drugs online if they searched hard enough. Keeping teens' social media and gaming accounts private (see "Practical Takeaway" box on pages 319–320) can also prevent them from being contacted by drug dealers.

Risky Sexual Contact

Risky sexual contact can include several situations.

- **Unwanted sexual solicitation:** This refers to when anyone known or not known to your child reaches out online and tries to get them to engage in sexualized communication. This can happen over text, messaging platforms, gaming platforms, or social media. This communication could include sending photos, talking to them online about sex or sexual situations, or even trying to meet in person. A 2018 study combined data from studies over almost 2 decades to better understand this experience, and the investigators found that about 11% of youth experience unwanted sexual solicitation online.

- **Sexting:** Sexting is sending, receiving, or forwarding sexually explicit messages, photographs, or videos using technology. It can include images of nudity or images that are sexually suggestive, such as photos of cleavage or people dressed in sexy outfits. A 2025 study in *Computers and Human Behavior* found that about 12% of youth had sent a sext willingly, and 4.1% of youth had sent a sext under pressure.
- **Sextortion:** This newer term describes when someone manipulates, coerces, or threatens a person into providing sexually explicit images or videos. This situation often happens when a teen is approached via social media or on a gaming platform by a profile that appears to be another teen. Usually, it starts with flirting and progresses to being asked to provide sexy or nude photos. Once the photos are sent, the person reveals themselves to be an adult and asks for money. If money is not sent, the person typically threatens to share the photos with the teen's family, friends, school, or community. There have been several high-profile and utterly tragic cases in which a teen lost their life to suicide due to the stress and danger of sexploitation. A 2024 international study of people of all ages published in *Computers and Human Behavior* found that about 14.5% of participants reported being victimized, and 4.8% of participants reported acting as a perpetrator.

As a parent you may be saying, "Whoa, not my kid!"

We get it. We all want to think that our own kids will be safe from sexual predators. We also want to think that our kid would never send a sext and would know exactly what to do if they are the 1 in 4 kids who will receive a sext at some point. How do we keep them safe and provide them with a sense of what to do in dicey situations? You guessed it—provide education and ongoing discussion on these tricky topics. We share strategies for talking with your child about sexting in Chapter 4.

Prevention: How to Set Up Healthy Media Boundaries

At this point you may be thinking, "How can I prevent my child from ever seeing this content?"

We agree—it is very hard to protect your child from ever seeing a representation of substance use, online challenges, gambling, or risky sexual content in media. The good news is that there are resources you can use when your child is younger to help navigate this situation. When your child is older, they may find this content either intentionally or unintentionally, and media can present you opportunities as a parent to have teachable moments.

It Starts With You

Parents may want to start by checking their own social media use. Are drug-related, violent, dehumanizing, or sexualized videos showing up in your feed? If yes, you can report, block, or click the "I'm not interested" button to hide or avoid these videos, giving them less attention overall. Talk to your kids while making these decisions to role model critical thinking and impulse control.

Young Children

Avoid normalization of sassy, sexualized, or violent challenges by monitoring (or avoiding) YouTube. We know this is a tough one! Many children love YouTube. But challenges show up in a lot of "kidfluencer" content, pranks particularly, so if you see your child watching these, talk about any behavior you see as not OK. You can also block the channel where the sassy or pranking behavior occurs.

Parents can also use the Common Sense Media resources to actively evaluate the content that young kids consume. This approach can help you limit exposure to health risk behavior content. Its lists of TV and movies include specific designation of whether the content includes substance use, violence, or sexual content. As kids get older, parents can ask their kids to look up the content themselves and see if it passes the test.

If your child is exposed to content about any of these risk behaviors, it is common for them to have questions about it. Parents may be tempted to say, "That is for adults," and stop there. We encourage you to go a step further to consider sharing *why* (remember, autonomy support involves providing the rationale for limitations). For example, if your child is exposed to funny content about substance use, try saying, "This is a substance that is for adults because it can do harm to your brain while your brain is still growing." Your child may have questions about the differences among substances such as alcohol, tobacco, or illegal drugs. Answer honestly and to the best of your knowledge, and, if appropriate, you can look online together to find answers. It's also OK to share your family, cultural, or faith or belief values with your child at these ages to help frame how your family approaches that type of substance use.

Elementary School and Middle School Years

For older children, parents can co-view content when possible. Content including references to substance use or sexual topics presents an opportunity to have a discussion with your child. Keep in mind that parents often say that talking with their kids about substance use and about sex are 2 of the toughest topics to bring up and talk about without running the risk of sounding like they are giving a lecture. A media representation of either of these topics is a great starting point, allowing you to ask questions such as "What did you think of how that story was told?" Another question to consider asking older children is "How did that story make you feel about that behavior?" This approach offers an opportunity to allow your child to share how they are thinking about what they saw. It also offers the opportunity for parents to correct any misinformation or misinterpretations and to show that having an open dialogue about these tough topics is healthy and normal.

Adolescents

During the teenage years, youth have much more independence with their media content. There is also a lot of media geared toward teens that makes substance use funny or cool. Parents may remember movies from their youth, such as *Animal House*, *Superbad*, or *Can't Hardly Wait*, or any of those coming-of-age movies that included teens using alcohol, tobacco, or drugs or seeking to have risky sex. Co-viewing content with teens to understand what they are seeing is important. It is a different strategy at this age, and you may need to hold your breath watching content that is unrealistic, silly, or clearly not targeted to parents. Understanding what kind of media your teen is interested in allows you the opportunity to have those follow-up conversations. Certainly, it is OK to place boundaries around content that doesn't align with your family rules. Some families base rules on movie and TV ratings, and others place rules about specific content such as substance use, violence, or sexual content. During adolescence, teens need to know exactly what the rules are and why they exist. Since teens spend time at friends' houses, it's important to discuss how and whether rules apply there. If your teen is at a friend's birthday party and they are going to watch *Superbad*, does that mean they need to come home? Be clear and involve your child in shaping how the rules work and where. You'd better be able to do this with an understanding of the range of content they engage in often and by inviting them to be part of setting the rules.

Conversation Tips | **Risky Behaviors**

I (Megan) remember a patient whose mom was concerned that her son was really into watching a show that included a storyline about drug use. She had a close friend who had died of an overdose and did not want him exposed to this show. She was worried that it would glorify drug use or get him interested in trying drugs. I initially suggested co-viewing the show, but she felt so sad about her friend who had died that she did not feel comfortable watching the show with him. Wow, that is valid. She wasn't sure how to talk about her concerns with her son. After discussing this dilemma, she decided that she would share these exact thoughts and feelings with her son. She explained that she understood he was interested in and excited about the show, and she shared her concerns and sadness about losing her friend. Her son was initially a little taken aback; "It's just a show, Mom," was an initial reaction. But when he saw her feelings and how much she missed her friend, they had an honest conversation about what they each felt about drug use. This allowed the mom to share advice and values with her son in a way that meant more to her son because now he knew and understood her experiences.

Prevention: How to Navigate Risky Online Behaviors

Online Gambling

It's important to teach your teens to understand the risks of compulsive gambling and losing money. I (Jenny) recently listened to the *Against the Rules* podcast (season 6) with my sons about the history of sports betting legalization, how statistically likely it is that people will lose bets, and the real-life effects of gambling on families. Teens have a pretty strong sense of fairness, and my boys were appalled to learn that users are regularly enticed to bet on parlays—the type of bets that almost always lose you money and thus make the app money. We also talked about the fact that college sports players experience harassment online from strangers who bet and lost on their performance in a particular game. Both of my boys love sports, so the idea of soccer games, basketball games, or a swimming race being tainted by the toxicity of people who are desperate because they lost money was a real turnoff to them.

Another way to build up some critical resistance to online gambling is to talk to your kids about any people you know who may have lost a lot of money gambling and how this affected them. For example, if you have a friend or family member who went through rough times, such as a divorce or losing their house, because they lost money on gambling, talk about it with empathy. This humanizes the issue by making it real and not just a shiny commercial where it looks like everybody wins.

As always, manage or monitor your child's app downloads to prevent them from using betting programs. Avoid apps that are like casino games, which include a lot of gambling elements but without the payout.

Video Games That Simulate Online Gambling

Become familiar with the video games your child plays. Play along, and see what type of pressure to encourage purchases exists in the game. If gambling-type designs are used, talk about how it feels to anticipate the unlocking and then the rush of excitement or disappointment that can follow. Kids often need help building insight into these emotional reactions to technology design.

Using gaming parental controls, put weekly or monthly spending limits on your child's or teen's account. Fortnite didn't have this type of parental control until they were sued by the Federal Trade Commission in 2023. Consider not including a credit card in the account until you have approved the game they would like to purchase.

If you don't like the gambling-type designs of games your child plays, talk about what other games they could play—maybe ones with more strategy or excitement built into the gameplay. Conduct an experiment to see whether switching to a game without gambling-like designs leads to less spending and more saving of their hard-earned allowance.

What to Do When You See Risky Content

It's Friday night, and your teen has agreed to watch a movie with you. You pick one of your old favorites from when you were a teen. You are so excited to be watching with your teen, but suddenly…halfway through the movie…you realize there is a scene that clearly includes health risk behaviors or problematic messages. When I (Megan) watched *Sixteen Candles* with my daughter, there were *a lot* of scenes that had not aged well. In particular, there was a scene involving sexual contact with someone who was too drunk to give consent. That was awkward. I ended up pausing the movie for a minute to acknowledge how weird I felt having been so excited to watch this movie with my daughter and then have that kind of story show up. We talked for a couple minutes about what story that scene was telling, and I shared that I hadn't really remembered that part and why that may be. I asked if she wanted to keep watching, and we finished the movie. Afterward, we talked about several of the storylines and what we each thought of them. We talked about how we sometimes watch movies that include stories we wouldn't want to happen to us (or anyone else) and what exactly we are supposed to learn from that.

I still felt kind of uneasy about that situation, but by my being open to asking how she felt, my daughter felt heard. I hope that talking about how media can show you stories, relationships, and communication that you would never want in real life can be a teacher. Just not the only teacher.

Content Blockers and Monitoring Apps

Although many parents wish there was a way to completely and accurately block sexual or risky content from reaching their child, or to monitor their child's media consumption to flag if they are exposed to this content, this still would not prevent all exposure. Software and blockers can often remove or lower the risk of exposure to the most extreme or obvious sexual content, but they cannot protect your child from what they may see on a friend's phone or a cousin's tablet. They can't protect them from media narratives that depict pushing for sex in unwanted situations, unprotected sex, or partners being unkind. As a parent, you can talk with your child about relationships that are based on respect, partnership, and kindness and remind them that media stories often show things that are rare or scary or for dramatization.

Practical Takeaway | **Preventing Risky Content and Contacts**

Every device that your child or teen has access to should have some type of filter or parental control to ensure that inappropriate content and contact are minimized. Here's how.

- Use the child's real age. Any devices, gaming platforms, streaming video or music, or social media should know your child's real age. Tell your kids that falsifying their age online might be easy, but it opens them up to scammers and harmful content.
- Use your home Wi-Fi controls to filter out pornography and other inappropriate content on all devices. Content filters are also standard on Apple and Android devices under family settings. (See the Resources for Parents for updated lists of parental controls).
- Set all child and teen accounts to private to prevent contact from predators, scammers, and drug dealers.
- Set download controls, particularly for children and younger teens. You will still want to monitor what your older teen downloads or purchases, but give them more independence based on their track record of good judgment. This is one way to keep AI chatbots and unsafe chat platforms off your child's device.

- Set purchase limits on gaming, social media, and app stores so that you can monitor and limit purchases. This will give you insight into whether your child is trying to purchase loot boxes or other risk-based rewards frequently. (It's also OK to set purchase limits to $0 and tell your kids that in-game purchases are off-limits.)

If your child or teen is more of a risk-taker who struggles to follow technology limits, take it slow with getting their first smartphone, social media account, or video games with gambling-like elements.

Remember, any parental controls and settings need to be combined with conversations so that you can monitor your child's digital life. Here are some general questions that you can use to touch base about risky content online.

"I keep seeing ads for [name of risky product]. Are you seeing those too? What do you think?"

"What is the creepiest thing that showed up in your feed this week?"

"Why do you think [risky activities] are so appealing to teens? Do you see other kids using these?"

Talking to Your Child About Risky Sexual Contact

A key finding in the many research studies about sexting and unwanted sexual solicitation is that parents who incorporate 2 strategies have kids who do OK navigating these scary situations. The first strategy involves parents talking to their kids to define what sexting and unwanted sexual solicitation are and ways to be careful. The other strategy is having parents tell their kids that they can come to them for support if this happens. These are the 2 most critical messages you can provide your child.

Unwanted Sexual Solicitation

Define what this is with your child (see page 312). Then talk through some strategies with them.

- If the person is unknown to you or your child, do not respond. Block them. If this occurs on social media platforms where you can take further action, report the message.

- If the person is known to you or your child and the person is an adult, do not respond. Talk with your children to figure out a strategy, which may involve reporting the message, blocking the person, or connecting to law enforcement.
- If the person is known to you or your child and the person is a teen, there are a couple strategies you can take. One is to try to deflect the message with humor—something like "You know I wouldn't do that, so why are you even asking?" If the message is more offensive or the person is not a close peer, consider not responding to it and then blocking future messages. If the contact is persistent, you may consider involving the teen's parents or potentially asking the school to be involved if the person is also interacting with your child at school.
- In all cases described here, save the messages or take screenshots in case it becomes more of a problem.

Sextortion

When talking about this with your child, discuss the risks of being approached online or on social media by strangers who appear to be teens but who may not be teens. This communication often happens in private messages within social media but could happen via chat, texting, or even email. The communication may start out as friendly messages or compliments on your child's appearance or personality. Over time, sometimes a matter of days or weeks, the messages usually shift to asking for more information about your child (eg, Where do they live? Who are their best friends? What school do they go to?). Then comes the ask for a nude photo.

The most common situation we hear about in the media is when a child sends a nude photo to someone posing as an adolescent and then that person becomes a blackmailer. This means that the person says that the teen has to give money or the blackmailer will share the nude photo with friends, family, school, or the community.

An important message to provide your child, knowing how scary and embarrassing these situations can be for teens, is that *you are there to support your child no matter what happens or how far a given situation may go.* The blackmailer is to blame, not your child. Even if they regret their actions, what the blackmailer is doing is a crime. For tech-savvy teens who are used to navigating online and meeting new people, this message may need to be discussed on multiple occasions.

The following tips are ways to help:

1. Report the account and situation to the platform immediately.
2. Block the blackmailer but do not take down your teen's profile, as sometimes it can be used by law enforcement or the platform to locate the blackmailer.
3. Use resources to help remove images (if they are sent out online), including the following:

    a. The National Center for Missing & Exploited Children (NCMEC): www.missingkids.org/gethelpnow/isyourexplicit contentoutthere

       This website provides information about how to report the incident and offers information on next steps you can take to protect your child from further distribution of the photo.

    b. Take It Down: https://takeitdown.ncmec.org

       This organization is dedicated to helping victims of sextortion find and take down online photos.

If you are considering sending money, keep in mind that this action usually just delays the release of the photos and leads to additional requests and escalation of blackmail. If you are unsure of whether to send money, consult with law enforcement or an expert at NCMEC before doing so. If your child already sent money and there are repeated requests for money, do not send additional money.

Connecting the Dots

Risk-taking is a developmentally expected behavior that peaks in adolescence. Help your child understand and avoid risky content and contacts; preventive approaches and regular conversations are key ways to reduce their risks while keeping your relationship healthy as they build their independence. Maintain a mindset that you can learn about online risks together, and help your teen know that you come from a place of loving protection rather than control.

- **Have a family conversation about online and offline risks:** Which ones are harder to avoid? Are pressures to be cool, strong, brave, or sexy more intense in person (eg, at school or during sports) or online? Where are you more likely to encounter creepy adults—offline or online? Listen to your kids' experiences of which risks are easiest to avoid versus most tempting to join in.
- **Talk to your friends:** Consider talking to your friends about some of the movies, shows, and media that you grew up with and what messages about sex were in those stories. Ask your parent friends how they handle talking to their own kids about risky sexual content in movies, and be open to sharing your wins and losses in your conversations with your own kids. Normalizing this topic and leaning into friends can be helpful in handling the awkwardness together.

FINAL CONNECTIONS

You are now at the end of the book. Thanks for joining us on this journey of connecting! Here are a few things that we hope you will take away from reading this book.

- **Technology, digital media, and screen time don't occur in a vacuum.** There are many factors, including our stress levels, the availability of child care or after-school programs, or a family's communication patterns that influence how technology is used and what affect it has on us.
- **Parenting around technology is not easy.** There are issues that make it harder, including polarization concerning this topic (Tech is only bad! Tech is only good!); competition among and between parents; and navigating the ever-changing world of technology with new devices, platforms, games, and tools.
- **There is more than one right way to parent around technology.** It's OK for your child to make mistakes, and for you to make mistakes, and to learn from them together.
- **Secure relationships form the bedrock of child and adult mental health.** When you find yourself in doubt with a decision related to parenting around technology, you can come back to key concepts, including how to support relationships; avoid power struggles; and carve out time for family, peers, and offline experiences.

When we are more aware of these factors, we can move away from immediately blaming ourselves when our family is struggling with tech use—and the emotions that self-blame can evoke. Instead, we can adopt a more practical mindset that prioritizes 2 core things. The first is **relationships**—connecting with our family, asking questions about how kids *and* parents are experiencing new technologies, and thereby building habits of regular communication and critical thinking about the digital world and how it supports or undermines our well-being. The second is **boundaries.** In a digital world that makes money off of people's time and attention, the best way to feel in control is to preserve spaces and daily routines that don't involve tech (or that use tech in a relationship-centered way). We've reviewed a lot of ways to do this, from everyday moments like car rides to bedtime strategies to movie nights, to intentionally setting up offline activities that meet your child's drives to connect socially, explore their sense of self, and meaningfully engage in the world.

What's Next?

You live a busy life, so we wrote this book to be read in bite-size amounts that you can try to apply to everyday life. Key topics and principles are **bolded** throughout the book. Also, if your child has questions or you want some advice on a particular issue, such as influencers, parental controls, or misinformation, you can look it up in the index, which provides links to those sections in the book.

We shared in the Introduction that we want this to be a book that you can refer back to as your child grows older or struggles with new things. Keep it on your bookshelf so that you can check back in as your child reaches milestones, like getting their first phone or first social media account. Our goal is to help you navigate and learn from these new milestones, which is what we as parents do across so many aspects of our children's lives. Thank you for joining us and being part of the good enough parent community around connecting.

RESOURCES FOR PARENTS

General Resources for Healthy Technology Use and Emotional Well-Being

The American Academy of Pediatrics Center of Excellence on Social Media and Youth Mental Health: 5 Cs of Media Use

www.aap.org/5Cs

This resource features videos, handouts, and other resources that provide ideas for healthy boundaries around media.

The American Academy of Pediatrics Family Media Plan

www.healthychildren.org/English/fmp/Pages/MediaPlan.aspx

This plan has several sections that can help specifically with promoting healthy sleep. These include setting media time limits in the Media Balance section and considering screen-free zones or screen-free times. The Choosing Good Content section could be used to select content you will focus on near bedtime to promote calm and winding down the day.

Common Sense Media

www.commonsensemedia.org

This website allows you to search types of media, such as gaming, social media, and movies. For each game or movie or platform, it describes the types of content a viewer may see, including content related to violence and aggression. It also has a section focused on "ultimate guides" for parents about video games, social media, AI, and parental controls.

Users can subscribe to newsletters and access several reviews for free before needing to create a paid account.

Harvard Center for Digital Thriving

https://digitalthriving.gse.harvard.edu/resources

This research and education center provides youth-centered and thoughtful, creative guidance on how to have healthy relationships with technology.

NetFamilyNews: Parenting Blog

www.netfamilynews.org/category/parenting

This website translates research and news into tips and information for families.

Mental Health and Emotional Well-Being

American Academy of Child and Adolescent Psychiatry: Facts for Families Guide: www.aacap.org/AACAP/Families_and_Youth/Facts_for_Families/Layout/FFF_Guide-01.aspx

This website provides lots of easy-to-understand resources for parents about different mental health conditions.

PBS for Parents: Emotions & Self-Awareness

www.pbs.org/parents/learn-grow/all-ages/emotions-self-awareness

These videos and resources provide ideas for development of emotional skills, using PBS characters.

Sesame Workshop: Emotional Well-Being

https://sesameworkshop.org/topics/mentalhealth

Sesame Street resources for families to support emotional development in young children. This includes videos with favorite characters, coloring pages, and ideas for parents.

Mental Health America

https://mhanational.org

Mental Health America is a nonprofit organization that has resources for youth and adults about understanding mental illness, crisis services, and building resilience.

The Jed Foundation

https://jedfoundation.org/mental-health-resource-center

https://jedfoundation.org/help-my-teen-young-adult

The Jed Foundation focuses on prevention of suicide and offers lots of resources for parents to understand how to help their teen.

The National Alliance on Mental Illness (NAMI)

www.nami.org

NAMI has resources about different aspects of mental health conditions, supports, and how to get support.

The Trevor Project

www.thetrevorproject.org

www.thetrevorproject.org/resources

The Trevor Project provides resources for youth, parents, and allies of LGBTQAI+ individuals to help support mental health and prevent suicide.

Zero to Three

www.zerotothree.org/resource/tips-for-promoting-social-emotional-development

These resources provide practical ideas for how to promote social-emotional development in early childhood, which lays the foundation for later mental health and social skills.

The Zones of Regulation

www.zonesofregulation.com

The Zones of Regulation curriculum and posters provide a color-coded visual guide for young children and their parents to name and manage different emotions.

Book: *The Explosive Child* by Ross Greene

https://drrossgreene.com/the-explosive-child.htm

Learn about the concept of a child's lagging skills, how to support them, and how to avoid power struggles with *The Explosive Child* by Ross Greene.

Substance Use

The National Institute on Drug Abuse (NIDA) and National Institute on Alcohol Abuse and Alcoholism (NIAAA)

https://nida.nih.gov and www.niaaa.nih.gov

These sites provide information and resources for parents and include information about the effects of substances on the brain and body and answers to frequently asked questions.

The Substance Abuse and Mental Health Services Administration (SAMHSA)

www.samhsa.gov

This site includes prevention sections specifically for parents and caregivers, including strategies about how to talk with your child about alcohol and other substance use.

Teen-Directed Health Resources

Susan Crown Exchange: Digital Well-Being

www.youthdigitalwellbeing.org/do

www.youthdigitalwellbeing.org/resources

These resources were supported by a collaboration involving the Susan Crown Exchange and provide a learning hub focused on thriving youth in a digital world.

American Academy of Pediatrics: After Hours Health

This site is focused on teen health and providing accurate information from pediatricians and other health professionals, along with youth experts, who get that health info doesn't have to be boring, confusing, or packed with scary medical terms.

Health for Teens

www.healthforteens.co.uk

Health for Teens is a great UK-based resource that provides information about different health conditions, mental well-being, and sexual health for teen readers.

Planet Puberty

www.planetpuberty.org.au

Planet Puberty is an Australia-based resource that provides information about puberty for parents and teens with intellectual disability and autism.

Planned Parenthood

www.plannedparenthood.org/learn/teens/resources-for-teens

The Planned Parenthood site has a lot of resources for teens about respectful romantic relationships and sexual health and also includes links to other reliable accurate sources.

Healthy Teen Relationships

Northwest Portland Area Indian Health Board: Relationships & Dating

https://wernative.npaihb.org/my-relationships/relationships-dating/abuse-violence

A teen-focused website on healthy dating and romantic relationships.

NewYork-Presbyterian Hospital Center: Addressing Toxic Relationships

www.nyp.org/youthmentalhealth/toxic-relationships

This resource includes a mental health video for teens on recognizing and addressing toxic relationships.

Love Is Respect

www.loveisrespect.org

This is a great website for teens that teaches about setting healthy boundaries, ending unhealthy relationships, and other important topics.

Sleep

B-SATED Research Article

The following is the research article that describes the B-SATED model created by sleep researchers Drs Meltzer, Williamson, and Mindell: www.sciencedirect.com/science/article/abs/pii/S1087079221000101

National Sleep Foundation: Teen Sleep Toolkit

www.thensf.org/teen-sleep-toolkit

This site focuses on helping teens get healthy sleep.

The Pediatric Sleep Council

https://babysleep.com

This website has resources focused on helping your child aged 0 to 3 years get better sleep.

Problematic Media Use

AAP Center of Excellence on Social Media and Youth Mental Health: Problematic Media Use Resources

www.aap.org/en/patient-care/media-and-children/center-of-excellence-on-social-media-and-youth-mental-health/problematic-media-use-screening-and-intervention-tools-for-clinicians

This page focuses on problematic media use and provides a summary of what it is, screening tools, prevention tips, interventions, and resources. While the page was created for clinicians to use in working with patients and families, the information can also be used by families.

Physical Activity, Outdoors, and Community Activities

Afterschool Alliance

www.afterschoolalliance.org

This organization promotes available activities for kids to engage in after school through research, funding, education, and resource sharing.

Boys & Girls Clubs of America

www.bgca.org

The Boys & Girls Clubs has connected youth to each other and activities for decades. Its website provides links to clubs and activities near you.

California Partners Project: Family Guide for Outdoor Movement

www.calpartnersproject.org/techlifebalance/movement

This resource provides practical, family-tested ideas for getting kids moving and outdoors.

HealthyChildren.org Fitness

www.healthychildren.org/English/healthy-living/fitness/Pages/default.aspx

This resource on HealthyChildren.org features several articles on how to fit physical activity into your day as well as different ideas for getting kids active.

Montefiore Health System: Teen Physical Activity Resources

https://montefioreeinstein.org/documents/catch/CATCH-Exercise-Teen-Physical-Activity-Web.pdf

This resource provides a worksheet of physical activity websites for teens.

YMCA

www.ymca.org

The YMCA has been around for 175 years and provides offline connection opportunities through classes and camps as well as ways to learn, move, and be connected.

Nemours TeensHealth: Physical Activity Guide

https://kidshealth.org/en/teens/center/fitness-nutrition-center.html

This resource offers youth a physical activity guide.

Body Image

The National Eating Disorder Association (NEDA): Body Image

www.nationaleatingdisorders.org/body-image

This website provides resources on body image.

The Body Positive

https://thebodypositive.org/5-competencies

This nonprofit organization provides resources on competencies in developing a positive body image.

Artificial Intelligence

Brookings Institution: "Tips for Parents: Raising Resilient Learners in an AI World"

www.brookings.edu/articles/tips-for-parents-raising-resilient-learners-in-an-ai-world

This article helps provide insight into possible negative effects of AI on youth learning, what parents can do about this, and how to raise AI-resilient learners.

Online Gambling

The Child Mind Institute

https://childmind.org/article/teens-and-online-gambling

This resource provides articles and parenting support about a range of child mental health issues, including this article on teens and online gambling.

Podcast: *Against the Rules*

Listen and learn about sports betting and mobile gambling in the *Against the Rules* podcast (season 6) with Michael Lewis: www.pushkin.fm/podcasts/against-the-rules

Parasocial Relationships

Children's Mercy Hospital: "Understanding Parasocial Relationships in Teen Media Use"

www.childrensmercy.org/parent-ish/2026/02/parasocial-relationships

An article written by Dr Libby Milkovich describing benefits, risks, and strategies around teen parasocial relationships.

Center for Scholars & Storytellers at UCLA: "You've Got a Friend in Me—The Benefits of Parasocial Relationships"

www.scholarsandstorytellers.com/blog/how-to-write-characters-who-connect-parasocial-relationships

An article on the benefits of parasocial relationships for young kids.

Violence and Bullying

National Domestic Violence Hotline

www.thehotline.org

This site includes web, chat, texting, and phone support for parents worried about their child or for teens themselves. This is a comprehensive resource focused on this topic area and is highly recommended.

Parent Tips on Virtual Violence and Kids from the American Academy of Pediatrics

www.youtube.com/watch?v=56qI3tBFrQ4

This video offers tips on how to prevent exposure to virtual violence and how to talk to your child if they are exposed to this content.

United Nations: "Hate Speech and Real Harm"

www.un.org/en/hate-speech/understanding-hate-speech/hate-speech-and-real-harm

This article describes the power of hate speech and how it is linked to violent actions in history.

The Conversation: "From Tarantino to Squid Game: Why Do So Many People Enjoy Violence?"

https://theconversation.com/from-tarantino-to-squid-game-why-do-so-many-people-enjoy-violence-170251

Why do people enjoy violent media? This article describes some potential explanations for why some people really enjoy media with stories that involve violence.

Cyberbullying Research Center

https://cyberbullying.org

This website has excellent content related to addressing sexting (and cyberbullying), including guidance on how to contact platforms and websites if your child's sexts ended up on social media.

Nutrition and Eating Disorder Prevention

The Society of Behavioral Medicine: Healthy Living

www.sbm.org/healthy-living/promoting-healthy-eating-habits-and-patterns-for-teens

This website provides ways to support healthy eating patterns for teens.

National Alliance for Eating Disorders: "'All Foods Fit' and Eating Freely in Eating Disorder Recovery"

www.allianceforeatingdisorders.com/all-foods-fit

This resource describes the "all foods fit" approach to reduce labeling of foods as "good" or "bad."

Sexual Exploitation

National Center for Missing & Exploited Children (NCMEC): Sextortion

www.missingkids.org/theissues/sextortion

This website provides information about sextortion and how to prevent and manage it.

Take It Down

https://takeitdown.ncmec.org

This service coordinates removing explicit images from websites and social media platforms and provides resources for parents on how to support their child through such an incident.

Parental Controls

InternetMatters.org provides a guide to available parental controls and privacy settings for child and teen devices: www.internetmatters.org/parental-controls

ConnectSafely has a Family Guide to Parental Controls: https://connectsafely.org/controls

Common Sense Media has a Parents' Ultimate Guide to Parental Controls: www.commonsensemedia.org/articles/parents-ultimate-guide-to-parental-controls

INDEX

Page numbers followed by *f* indicate a figure; by *t,* a table; and by *b,* a box.

P

S

Also Available From the American Academy of Pediatrics